Fit
for
God

Fit
for
God

The 8-Week Plan
that Kicks the Devil
Out and Invites
Health and
Healing In

La Vita Weaver

DOUBLEDAY

New York London Toronto Sydney Auckland

PUBLISHED BY DOUBLEDAY

a division of Random House, Inc.

DOUBLEDAY and the portrayal of an anchor with a dolphin are registered trademarks of Random House, Inc.

Book design by Chris Welch

Library of Congress Cataloging-in-Publication Data

Weaver, La Vita.

Fit for God : the 8-week plan that kicks the Devil out and invites health and healing in / La Vita Weaver.— 1st ed.

p.   cm.

1. Health—Religious aspects—Christianity.   2. Spiritual life.   I. Title.

BT732. W43 2004

248.4—dc22

2003055707

ISBN 0-385-49832-2

PRINTED IN THE UNITED STATES OF AMERICA

February 2004

3   5   7   9   10   8   6   4

Fit for God is dedicated to all of the wonderful people
in my life who have truly been with me on the journey of
my healing and deliverance:

The best mom in the world, Marcia Lawrence, for her
unconditional love, support, and godly wisdom; my stepdad,
Michael Lawrence, who has truly been a great father and an
awesome grandfather; my uncle Walter Weaver, "Uncle Henry,"
who has been a father, a big brother, and a best friend all in one;
my oldest brother, Arthur Weaver, Jr., for his words of wisdom and
encouragement; my pastor and sister, LaReese Brooks, who has
been my mentor, my confidante, and my best friend; my
brother-in-law, Ulysses Brooks, who has been a true brother
indeed; my younger brother, James, and his lovely wife, Thereasé,
for their love and support; my younger sister, La Vinia Weaver, for
her kind, gentle spirit and loving support; and my three beautiful
daughters, LaTicia, LaTrina, and LaTia, who have been my
greatest blessings on Earth.

In memory of the late Arthur L. Weaver, Sr.
1939–1992

And last but not least, I thank my husband, Roberto Smith,
for teaching me how to stand in the midst of my trials.

Acknowledgments

I thank my Lord and Savior, Jesus Christ, from the depths of my soul for giving me a brand-new life. I thank Him for giving me the peace, joy, and freedom that I never imagined. I am eternally grateful because He sacrificed His life so I could be healed from all my hurt and disappointment, and free to be what he created me to be—fit for God, spirit, soul, and body.

Contents

The
Battle

Chapter One

As a child I thought my father was the best-looking person in our family. Arthur Weaver, known as Art or Lawrence (his middle name) to his friends and family, had honey brown skin and hair the color of sand. He had a keen nose and small lips, and when the sun shone on his almond-shaped eyes I saw pools of light brown glimmering in the center of rust-colored circles. They were breathtakingly beautiful.

My siblings and I were an autumn-colored rainbow—tan, reddish brown, yellow, and dark brown. My two sisters looked like my father. I called my baby sister "Sunshine" because she was pale yellow. I used to show her off to people and say, "Isn't she cute?" Everyone on television was white and most of my dolls were white. Everywhere I looked the world seemed to be saying, "White is the only color that is beautiful." And my father was the closest thing to white I had. I was the darkest girl in my family. My hair was short because of a nervous condition. I had a small nose, but it wasn't as narrow as my father's, and my wide lips came from my mother's broader features. It was okay for boys to be darker because they could still get what they wanted out of life, but everyone knew girls were supposed to be pretty and look a certain way. I figured I was destined to have a hard time in life.

The only things I had going for me were that I was athletic and that I was an honor roll student, both of which made me very popular in school.

In 1968, when I was five years old, we moved from our neighborhood in Washington, D.C., to a suburban community in Seat Pleasant, Maryland, following hundreds of other black working-class families who moved into houses originally built for white people. Our house was a two-story redbrick with a fence around the yard.

The county to which we moved had just started a new desegregation plan, busing white students into what had been a predominantly black elementary school. I was placed in the advanced classes, where most of the students were white. A white girl named Nancy became my best friend, and sometimes I went home on weekends with her. But in general there was friction between many of the black kids and white kids.

My black classmates thought I should choose either black friends or white ones, because it was impossible to have both.

"Vidi, you act like you think you're white," they said over and over.

I didn't care, though, because my white friends treated me better than my black classmates did. My white friends didn't care that my hair wasn't long, that I wore glasses, or that my skin was dark. I earned their respect because I was always on the honor roll.

The taunts from black students increased.

"You think you're too good for us?" they hollered.

"You need to hang with your own kind!"

I was shorter than most of them, but I really wasn't scared. I just didn't want to fight. My older sister, LaReese, however, insisted, "Vidi, if you run they'll never stop."

So it was inevitable that one day I had to face my taunters. As I approached the group, a girl with an irritating, high-pitched voice said, "Look who's coming."

I slowed down and stood in front of her with my arms folded. She pushed me. I pushed back. We tussled and the next thing I knew I was pulling her hair and scratching her and she was screaming. We rolled around on the grass. Kids hollered and cheered.

Somebody broke us up. I checked my hair and clothes and found that my opponent had barely touched me but that her face was all scratched up. I walked away as the crowd parted.

I never had to run or avoid anyone again.

I am the middle child of five. I have a brother and sister older than me and a brother and sister younger than me. Our house was always busy, bursting with sound. A radio or stereo would play nonstop because my parents loved music and loved to dance. They would hand-dance in the middle of the floor, my father sliding his feet across the floor, twirling my mother. Then she'd stop quickly and ease into step with him, matching his rhythm. We kids would sit watching, oohing and aahing at their coolness, and then we would clap enthusiastically at the end of the song.

In the evening and on weekends my father and brothers cheered and hollered as they tossed a football to each other. Sometimes my father stood in the middle of the street and threw long arching balls that landed right at the chest of one of my brothers, who then ran around the yard boasting.

We had a lot of family gatherings: crab feasts, fish fries, cookouts. My father brought home live crabs by the bushel and then poked at them as we watched, amazed and respectful of the big claws that grabbed at anything. My aunts, uncles, cousins, and Mama and Daddy's friends came to our cookouts and stuffed themselves and drank until some of them got real quiet while others got real loud.

Mother stayed home with us children while my father worked full-time as a mechanic at a car dealership and part-time driving a truck. He was proud that he was able to make enough money to take care of all of us. We had everything we needed and most of what we wanted. We had the latest toys. I had Baby Tender Love, the first doll to look like a real baby with white, soft skin, blue eyes, and blond hair. As I got older I collected Barbies. I had a dollhouse with more furniture in it than we had in our house.

Little creatures just fascinated me. I had dogs, cats, turtles, hamsters, gerbils, and fish. My brother Lawrence used to go fishing in my fish tank with a needle and thread. Generally he wanted to help and protect us, which is why he dreamed of becoming a superhero. It made sense later that as an adult he became a police officer.

The three oldest of us used to play church a lot, which is fitting now too because we are all ministers today. Church was a big part of our life. My family, minus my father, went to Carmody Hills Baptist Church, faithfully. As far back as I can remember I went to Sunday school and church service almost every Sunday.

My father was well liked by everyone because he kept people laughing. He was handsome, youthful, energetic, and athletic. He never looked his age. He was a good father and he enjoyed being one, spending a lot of time camping and fishing with his boys. Our life was carefree and full of fun and people and laughter.

Then one day when something horrible happened and we all changed forever. That day is a bookmark in my life. There is life before it and the pages of life lived after it.

I was in third grade and came home from school expecting nothing unusual. Mother was home as always, but it was strangely quiet. I do not remember whether or not Lawrence and LaReese were already there when I got home. What I remember is Mother taking the three of us to her bedroom and sitting with us on the bed.

"Your daddy has been in a terrible accident at work," she said, her lips trembling. "He was in a fire. He was burned pretty bad." Tears streamed down her cheeks. She paused and looked somewhere beyond us. "He's in a coma—and he may die."

The words seemed to tumble out of her mouth, one sentence after another, without any breath in between.

Later, we saw a news report on TV about the accident. They speculated that someone was smoking a cigarette and threw a butt near a gas tank at the car dealership. The tank exploded and Daddy was surrounded by fire. The only way to get out was to run through the flames. They said my father was completely on fire and that some coworkers rolled him on the ground to put out the flames.

For the next few days people came to our house to sit with Mother. At times there was crying and whispering. We children could not go to the hospital to visit him, so all I knew were the frightening things I overheard: "His breathing stopped once," and "They're going to operate to help his skin heal."

I walked around with a nervous feeling inside me, half living, never really able to have fun or to put all of my attention on any one thing because I was always thinking of my father.

We did not see him until he got out of the hospital six months later. He had light spots on him where his skin had changed milky white. He was blessed because he still had his ears, nose, and lips. He had his hair, and none of his features were deformed. His skin even healed pretty well. After a while people knew something was wrong with his skin, but they could not tell he had been burned.

Still, he was never the same. The father who came home to us from the hospital was not the father we sent off to work on the morning of the fire. And because he changed, we all changed. For instance, we never took photos after my father came home. I did not realize this for years, not until I was much older and went to search for a family album. I found two pictures taken prior to the accident, and even on those someone had used a blue ink pen to mark through my father's face. There was a two-tone photo of him and Mother, young and smiling, standing at their wedding ceremony. She had on a wedding gown and he had on a suit. And there was another picture of my father sitting with two of his brothers. They were smiling and he was faceless. My assumption was that someone in the family who was angry with him started tearing up old photos and crossing out his face. I never asked anyone or said a word about my findings. But more recently, I considered the possibility that my father, who hated the way he looked after the fire, may have ruined the photos himself. At any rate, I so desperately wanted family photos that I took those two pictures and for years kept them in my Bible for safekeeping.

Daddy started drinking right after he came home from the hospital. Maybe he was drinking before the fire, but we children had never seen evidence of it. Now everyone knew. He hid bottles of vodka in the sofa, under a mattress, or behind drapes. Much later in my life I would realize that I did the same thing with food that my father did with alcohol. I hid snacks, ate in private, and couldn't wait to leave work just so I could stuff myself with junk food.

I was terribly unhappy with my life then, and I am sure my father drank so he could tolerate life, too. But when he drank his temper flared, though he never raised his voice at me.

He had plenty to be angry about. I don't think he ever went back to the car dealership. He found and lost a series of jobs for years afterward. The laughter in our house was replaced by arguing between my parents. Daddy lashed out at Mother with words first; as time passed, he struck her with his fists or hands or whatever he could find. I hated to come home because I never knew whom I was going to get—the gentle, sober father or the violent, drunk one.

I used to tell myself Daddy was sick, so I never got angry with him. I didn't think the accident justified what he was doing, but I thought there was a demon inside him. The demon was just one part of him because another part of him remained the same. He and I still laughed and joked, and I still enjoyed him more than anyone else in the world. But his eyes could change and look eerie and distant, and you knew it was going to be a bad day. If he drank, he treated everybody badly except me and my younger brother and sister. Mostly he took his pain out on my mother and my older sister and brother.

My mother was pretty and dressed well, things Daddy found attractive before the accident. After the fire, he questioned her about everything. When she put on an outfit that used to be one of his favorites, he asked, "Why do you have to wear that?"

When he went drinking or gambling with his friends, I went with them, though my mother didn't want me to go. But my father, whose nickname for me was "La Vidi," just called to me and said, "La Vidi, get your coat," and I would be right beside him. When we got where we were going, if there were kids there I played with them. Otherwise, I just sat and watched my father.

God truly was with me. We were in a lot of car accidents. Sometimes the police brought me home because they were arresting Daddy.

We got used to the police coming to our house because my mother and father were fighting. I became an extremely private person because I didn't want to discuss my family life. When you have police and ambulances coming to your house regularly, you learn to keep quiet, even if you know that everyone else is gossiping about you.

My father collected guns and threatened to kill himself from time to time, so I watched him closely. One Saturday afternoon I left him to go to my room for a minute. I was not going to stay long because I knew Daddy had that eerie look in his eyes. Before I got back I heard a loud bang. I knew immediately what it was. I ran into the living room. Daddy was sitting on the sofa holding a shotgun in his hands. I sat down right next to him, maybe six inches away. I never feared my father, so even though he had a gun, I knew I was not in danger.

I did not realize it at the time, but my brother had seen my father with the gun and had run out of the house and to the police station a mile or so away. There are gaps in my memory about what happened that day.

I remember I left my father on the sofa long enough to peep out the window. I saw a lot of police officers with long guns jumping out of a truck and I thought: "This must be the SWAT team." But they didn't have to knock down our door like I had seen on television. Our door was unlocked, so the police just ran in, a whole, long line of them carrying guns.

Someone asked my father to put down his gun. And he did. I was still sitting right next to him and maybe that is what saved him from the police. An officer picked up the gun and found out it was empty. I have no recollection of what happened after the officer took the gun.

If Daddy started arguing in front of me, I tried to distract him with a temper tantrum or a request to go to McDonald's. Usually he stopped and gave in to me. It was so confusing to a child: A man who was loving and funny most of the time, then was crazy out of his mind the next minute.

My older sister and brother would not speak to him during this period. My nerves were so bad I pulled out my hair by the fistfuls and cut off my ponytails. I had short, uneven hair all the time. I bit my fingernails to the quick. The kids at school and even my sisters and brothers called me "bald-headed."

My mother encouraged me every way she could. "Vidi, you're just as pretty as anyone else. One day your hair is going to grow," she said.

We all hoped something dramatic and painless would happen to make my father stop drinking. But he kept it up. One time he had completely refinished the basement, working carefully and patiently for weeks on the walls. Then in a drunken flash he got mad and tore down every wall he had put up.

Finally, the year I went to junior high, my mother asked Daddy to move out. She called us children in to tell us he was gone. I ached all over, consumed by grief. I decided I could live with the pain of his being there, but I could not live with the hurt of him *not* being there.

To make up for my loss, I grabbed hold of my brother Lawrence, who was four years and three months older than me. He became the man I went to for advice, the one I ran to when I was proud of something I had done.

My father stopped coming by to visit. If I wanted to see him, I had to go wherever he was. He didn't give us any financial assistance either, so my mother got a job at the Bureau of Engraving, working twelve hours a day, seven days a week. Suddenly life had changed considerably because I seldom saw either of my parents.

We children went through a long period of being on our own. Yet nobody ran wild. We did our homework, honored our curfews, and kept the house clean. I felt as though I was the only one with problems. Inside, I was anxious, mourning all we had lost. It was only as an adult that I discovered that every one of my siblings was going through the same internal anguish. Yet each of us survived as best we could—in silence.

By this time I was beginning to look different. At thirteen, I developed a nice figure and started getting a lot of attention from boys. I ran track and was athletic, and my body showed it.

When I walked down the hall, guys made comments like "Oh my God, she's phat to death." They whistled, howled, whispered, and occasionally grabbed my arm. I loved to dance, and now all the boys wanted to dance with me. Sometimes I had to force them to keep a respectable distance.

I had always been popular in a way, mostly because of athletics and academics and because I was friendly. I won the Superintendent's Award, the highest academic award you could receive. I was a cheerleader for the county parks and planning department. But I had never received attention for my looks until the boys started calling out my name whenever I passed.

"Vidi, you know why those boys are looking at you, don't you?" my brother Lawrence asked me one day.

I was watching television and only halfway paying attention to him.

"They just want to sleep with you," he said. "They don't care about you, so don't get a big head."

I turned to look at him.

"Vidi, you know how precious and valuable gold is?" Lawrence asked. "Your body is like gold, and you don't give gold to anybody."

That got my attention, his comparing my body to gold. I made up my mind that I would have sex only after I got married.

I was in tenth grade when I met John, a twelfth grader at my school. Discovering that he liked me made me feel better about myself. To us girls, dating an older guy meant you were more of a woman. And John was cute and dressed as clean-cut and conservatively as I did. I wore business suits and dresses to school when other girls wore pants. I didn't wear a lot of makeup, and I wore dress pumps. John was my male counterpart. He wore suits also and, like me, it made him look older, more businesslike.

I went out on my first date—ever—with John. I had grown up with my mother drilling us girls, "Only have sex with your husband after you get married."

But John kept asking me. I said no, and we kissed. He asked again and we petted. He asked again, and I said no.

During my standoff with John, my brother Lawrence got married.

I was devastated. It seemed to me that he was leaving me just as my father had left. I cried during his wedding and for much of the reception.

I cannot say that Lawrence's leaving had anything to do with the turn in my relationship with John, but it all happened around the same time. John challenged me. "You're just scared to have sex," he said. I don't know why the challenge affected me the way it did, but I could never stand for someone to think I was scared of anything. I made an appointment to go over to his house to have sex while his mother was at work.

The night before I had a dream that God came to me. I heard Him clearly say that it was wrong to have sex, and if I did have it, I would regret it for a long time.

I told John about my dream; but he thought I was making it up, so we made another appointment. The night before that date, I had the same dream. I told John again, and again he said, "You're just scared."

"Maybe I *am* just scared," I said. I was definitely confused. And I was thinking to myself: Yeah, it is weird. God does not come to you in dreams. It must be my imagination.

So I had sex, but I did not really want to. I did it for the reasons a lot of young girls probably do, because you run out of ways to say no.

I knew what I had to do next: I told my mother. I could always talk to my mother about anything. I wasn't afraid of her. We always talked like girlfriends, maybe because in a way we grew up together. She grew into a new person without my father while I was growing from a girl to a woman. I will never forget the look of shock and disappointment on her face. She cried so much and when I tried to console her, I cried too.

She took me to the doctor, who confirmed what mother and I suspected: I was pregnant.

I felt as if I were dying. My life was slipping away. I think the reason none of us children had ever gotten into any real trouble was that we felt our mother had suffered enough and we wanted her to have an easier life now that my father was gone. And now I had hurt her.

She cried for days. I remember thinking: I'm *just* having a baby, and then I'm going to college.

Teachers had always described me as "gifted and smart" and said, "She is going to be somebody." My mother believed I would go straight from high school to greatness. All of her five children would do well, she was sure, but success for me had been a given. Until John.

Now she wanted a promise that I would finish high school. John endeared himself to her by saying he would make sure I graduated. Then he asked her if he could marry me. Considering the circumstances, he thought it was the right thing to do.

I didn't want to get married.

"If he loves you and you love him, Vidi, you should get married," Mama said.

I wanted a wedding, but we didn't have one because John was a Jehovah's Witness, which meant that if we had our ceremony at my church, his family would not be allowed to come. If I had the wedding at the Kingdom Hall, where his family worshiped, I would have to agree to raise the kids as Jehovah's Witnesses, and I didn't want to do that. So we just went to a justice of the peace with my mother and John's mother, a cousin, and an aunt. I wore a green maternity dress to hide my five months of pregnancy.

We had no honeymoon period, no peaceful period during which we could learn each other's habits. From the beginning my husband's jealousy caused me a lot of stress. In the midst of disappointment and failure, food became my comfort and friend.

I started snacking throughout the day, eating cookies, chips, cheese puffs, chocolate cupcakes, and ice cream. Eventually the small junk foods would no longer satisfy me, so I added larger portions of other fattening foods: pizza, steak, cheese subs, and items from fast-food restaurants. After every meal I ate another snack, and right before going to bed I ended my day with yet another. A nighttime snack for me was a whole pack of chocolate chip cookies and a sixteen-ounce glass of whole milk.

I was happy when I had food in my mouth. I got excited just planning the meal I was going to eat next.

During the nine months of my pregnancy I gained eighty pounds, almost ten pounds every month. The doctor was shocked and tested me to see if I was diabetic. Meanwhile, John enjoyed watching my petite figure disappear. Without my asking, he came home with pizzas, ice cream, and lots of milk. I drank a gallon of whole milk every two days.

I attended school until a few weeks before my due date. On December 3, 1980, I went into labor. As John sped through lights in his blue Volkswagen, I held my breath and gritted my teeth.

In the labor room at the hospital, John held my hand. The pain went on for hours. I listened to the loud beat of my baby's heart on the monitor. At one point the beat slowed. Then there was nothing. Silence. I was terrified. The nurses and doctors, who had been calm, now ran around frantically.

"Why, God, are you doing this?" I asked silently. "Am I being punished for having sex? Punish me, but don't punish my baby, please."

It was the worst moment of my life. Then I heard a faint heartbeat. They decided to give me a C-section, but I would not let them put me to sleep. I heard the heartbeat grow louder and stronger, and shortly afterward my baby was born.

It was a beautiful girl, eight and a half pounds. I let my eyes roll over every ounce of her: her chubby pie face, her jet black eyes, and her straight black hair. I counted her fingers and toes and then returned my eyes to hers. For a long time, it seemed there was no one else in the world at that moment except her—and me.

My husband was ecstatic, too. We named her LaTicia Maria.

When I left school to have my baby I had been a size 5, and when I returned I was a size 13. I still enjoyed running, but there was never enough time with a baby and a husband. I began taking diet pills. I needed a quick fix, a way to make the pounds fall off. I used the pills and prayed.

Somehow I managed to graduate from high school, though it was not the happy graduation day I had always envisioned. I was a wife and held a six-month-old baby in my arms. As friends left for college, a deep sadness covered me. I was angry and disappointed at myself.

Still, on graduation day I was hopeful that I would find a way to go to college. Once I got in college, everything would change, I told myself. It would be my victory, a way to prove to everyone—including myself—that I was not a failure.

Chapter Two

I planned to attend college when my daughter was older, and pursue my dream of becoming a doctor. But I married a man so jealous, he did anything he could to keep me dependent on him, and I was too young to fully understand what jealousy will make a person do.

John quit or got fired from every job he had, yet in the heat of arguments he yelled, "I want more children!" Two weeks after my high school graduation, I was pregnant again.

I felt as if someone had buried me alive. I struggled to breathe, a ton of weight on my chest. I kept my pregnancy a secret from everyone until my stomach told people the truth.

While I moped, barely able to get up and dress each day, John gloated and boasted.

"This is great, La Vita. We're going to have a *lot* of children—at least ten!" he shouted.

I cried, thinking about how often I was asking my mother for money to buy milk and diapers and to pay the electricity bill.

I got a temporary job with the post office, working the late shift, from 3 to 11 P.M. The bus didn't run at night, so I asked John to pick me up. He wanted me to stay home, so he made the job inconvenient for me. He picked me up but was always late, arriving after midnight when the building was locked and I was waiting outside alone.

"What kind of man do you have anyway?" male coworkers asked when they saw me standing outside.

"He gets off late sometimes," I answered.

It was easier to lie than to face the truth—that my husband was jealous and irresponsible.

I was afraid to eat during this pregnancy because I remembered my weight gain with my last baby. Most days I ate only one large meal a day at work—usually a sandwich or two and a salad with a snack. Still, I felt fat and was paranoid. When I went out in the public I thought everyone was staring at me.

I drank a lot of beverages. Whenever I felt my stomach rumble or felt hunger pangs, I drank soda, milk, Kool-Aid, or juice. At the time I didn't realize that those were high-calorie beverages. I thought I was avoiding calories.

In reality, I did not gain much at all for a pregnant woman, maybe twenty-five pounds during the entire nine months. Despite the reality, my paranoia about weight persisted. I stood in front of a mirror studying myself several times a day. I had a pair of pants I tried on regularly to see if I had gained.

I walked around hungry, but I didn't dare eat. Food meant fat to me. While I didn't physically crave food, I thought about it all the time because I was obsessive about not eating.

The lack of food seemed to make the baby move more. When I ate, the baby seemed to sleep well. I didn't worry about the baby's health because each time I went for a checkup the doctor said the baby was growing and everything was fine. Meanwhile, I seldom had a solid night's rest, but I shrugged that off to stress.

Somehow I maintained my sanity through those nine months, through arguments and periods when I couldn't buy diapers for my baby, and through the ups and downs of a relationship that bounced from laughter and fun to jealous rages and loneliness.

After nine months of stress and eating less, I gave birth to LaTrina, "my miracle child." I called her this because it was a miracle that she was perfect.

We moved back into my mother's house. John was unemployed again, and I resented him for that and for the imposition on my mother. I cried for long periods, depressed about how my life was unraveling.

I was always pleading, "John, I need some money for baby food. We're almost out of diapers."

"You can't squeeze blood out of a turnip" was his answer. "Besides, you know your mother wouldn't let you do without."

He counted on my mother's contribution to our budget the way people rely on a regular paycheck.

When I took the children to the doctor, we sat for hours in the emergency room with other people who had no health insurance. And when we finished, I received a hospital bill in my name.

I grew more and more depressed. I was nineteen years old, and while many of my friends were in college enjoying life and preparing for a better future, I had a fifteen-month-old baby, an infant, and an abusive, irresponsible husband. I felt my mind slipping away from me, separating me from reality.

I turned to food again. I ate, as before, because of stress and regret, but this time I also had a new companion—anger. I was angry with myself, angry with John. Whenever I was overwhelmed with anger, I went to the store and filled my basket with the goodies that calmed me: chocolate cookies, donuts, cheese puffs, and other snacks. Then I stuffed myself until I couldn't eat any more.

Soon I developed yet another habit. I felt so guilty after overeating that I took laxatives to rid myself of the food. Or I punished myself and tried to make up for the overeating by starving myself for a week. It wasn't long before this was a regular cycle. I overate, took laxatives, overate, and starved myself.

I was taking all of my anger and regret out on myself, and I couldn't stop. In the meantime I did everything possible to please John and let him know I was living in the Word, at least the way I understood it. I changed the way I dressed, making sure my clothes were not revealing. I tried harder than he did to make our marriage a success. In the end I stuck with him only because we had two children.

I was determined to hold on to my dream of going to college, though it might take me longer to get there. I decided to first go to business school at night to become a medical assistant, a stepping-stone to a better salary and, eventually, college. But John wouldn't babysit for me, so again I relied on my family. My mother and sister kept the children while I attended classes. John wouldn't even drop me off at school or at the subway station.

We argued constantly about his lack of work ethic and our lack of money. Finally one day I did the unthinkable: I applied for Aid to Families with Dependent Children, what people call welfare.

Walking into that welfare office was devastating for me. I was confessing publicly to strangers that I was a failure. The people who waited on me spoke to me with total disrespect.

"You're nobody and you'll never be nothing," John said to me all the time.

Now in one visit to a city office I was reduced to a statistic—a young black woman with babies.

My only comfort was my late-night snacking and bingeing. Food didn't talk back to me. Hostess Twinkies didn't put me down. Breyers ice cream didn't yell at me. Oreo cookies waited to give me pleasure.

My business courses made me believe I was moving forward. But after classes, I had to go home to my husband and the craziness that was growing worse.

One day I was walking down the street near my mother's house with one of my girlfriends and one of my cousins when John drove by. He and his friend Chris were looking for me. He had never met this cousin, so all he saw was me with a man. He backed up the car, stopped, and got out. He headed straight for my cousin.

"John, that's my cousin!" I screamed.

"Get in the car!" he ordered, his eyes wild and angry.

My girlfriend needed a ride, so she got in the backseat. When John stopped at my mother's, before I had even gotten out of the car, he was at the passenger door. He grabbed me by my throat with both his hands, choking me with all his strength. I gagged and fought. I gasped for breath. My girlfriend pulled him, but he wouldn't stop. Finally, Chris was able to restrain John.

I fell on my knees, gasping and coughing. My throat was raw. If the other two had not been there, he would have killed me, I was sure. I knew I would never trust John again.

"I want you out of here," I told him that night. "You've got to go!"

He left because he knew my mother would make him leave. I slept better that night than I had in weeks.

Without John, I truly had no source of income other than my family—and I still had no health insurance.

Because of the stress in my life, I continued my pattern of overeating and then fasting—going days without eating. My weight fluctuated up and down because of my eating habits. I ate my regular meals full of fattening foods, then finished it all off with high-calorie snacks. I craved sugar so badly that I started experimenting with different foods to find new ways of getting my fix. I made Pillsbury biscuits, loading them with butter and dipping them in King syrup. I ate all ten biscuits at one sitting. I made grilled cheese sandwiches, toasting them in a pan with lots of butter. Then I poured syrup over them, too. I saturated my ice cream with Hershey's chocolate and ate a row of Ritz crackers, each one loaded with cream cheese.

I ate until I was sick. Sometimes I automatically threw up, which was painful because the regurgitation made my stomach contract tightly, and that hurt. Occasionally I made myself throw up, but because of the severity of the pain I didn't do this often. I had to find another way to lose weight, so I started fasting and using diet pills regularly.

Eventually, after six months of fasting and dieting, I lost twenty pounds. This success changed my view of dieting or healthy eating. Regardless of how much I ate or what I ate, I now knew a sure way to shed pounds: All I had to do was fast. This pattern became my rhythm of life. I kept a closetful of clothes that included sizes 5, 7, and 9. I basked in the compliments from people who admired me for the weight I had lost. But there was no way I could maintain it.

I stepped into what today I call a body trap. I was trapped in my own flesh and its desires. I was out of control and saw no way out. And yet I remember telling my sister, "One day I'm going to write a book and tell people the way out."

The academic work still came easy for me, and studying was a way of mentally escaping the other part of my life. I graduated at the top of my class and had the highest test scores. I was proud of myself for the first time in years.

I got a job as a medical assistant/receptionist, aiding the doctor during physical examinations and routine laboratory work. John and

I rarely spoke. He saw the kids but did not pay child support. I fought him to get a legal separation and then finally a divorce. But whenever I asked him for money for the children, he'd tell me to ask my mother. *"You* decided to be single," he'd say.

My aunt sold me an old green Buick with a white vinyl top for five hundred dollars. Without John, I was very self-sufficient. I became the neighborhood hairstylist, earning extra money braiding and fixing hair.

But I was confused about God. Was He punishing me still for having gotten pregnant out of wedlock? Where I once had faith, now I worried about everything. What was going to happen to my children and me?

I did well on my job, but in the fall of 1984, I quit it to attend community college, still dreaming of a medical career. I worked a short while in a government job but was bored and miserable. My brother Lawrence was on the police force at the time, and what I noticed most was the satisfaction in his voice when he talked about police work. So I applied to the police department, took a test, and shortly afterward received a letter inviting me to enter the police academy. I was proud. As a result of the invitation, I quickly starved myself down to a size 5.

One day I was strolling through the mall, feeling good about myself and less burdened by the future, when I noticed this very good-looking guy staring at me.

"La Vita Weaver." He said my name as if he were delighted to see me.

I peered at him. Could it be Raymond Parker, my old friend and high school classmate? The Raymond Parker I remembered was a cute, scrawny kid, but this was a striking, pretty-boy type who could grace the cover of a magazine. Silky black hair, perfectly unblemished reddish brown skin, and big baby eyes with long eyelashes.

I was smitten from the beginning, mostly because of his good looks and his sense of humor, which reminded me of my father's. He kept me laughing—and I needed laughter.

He was well read. In fact, I met him in high school in the advanced placement classes. He was the kind of person everyone remembered fondly after just one meeting. Still, I got hints from the beginning that Raymond had issues he needed to deal with before he could be a healthy partner in a relationship. I chose to ignore those hints, perhaps the way I ignored them in the very first man I chose to love, my father.

Raymond was self-centered even when he was around my kids. *He* wanted the attention. He wanted his needs met before anyone else's. I constantly balanced giving him what he needed against not neglecting my kids.

Then his jealousy zoomed out of control and there was no denying it: Raymond was just like John, the husband I had escaped. At first Raymond seemed proud of my being in the police academy. But soon he made it obvious he was jealous of the other guys, my classmates. Our arguments grew more frequent and more violent, until he crossed the line and I knew my health would be in danger if I stayed with him.

We police cadets were having a graduation party. I asked Raymond to go with me, but he refused. He was so jealous of or intimidated by the other guys that he couldn't stand being with me around them. Since he would not go, I invited Nathan, a longtime childhood friend. But I didn't tell Raymond because I didn't want to argue.

As Nathan and I came out of the party that night, I saw Raymond drive up, his face distorted with rage and jealousy. He got out of his car and walked toward us.

"Let me go talk to him," I told Nathan, insisting he go sit in his car and wait.

I don't think I got a word out of my mouth before Raymond punched me so hard I hit the pavement and blacked out. Nathan jumped out of his car to chase him, but Raymond sped away. I tried getting up, but I was dizzy and disoriented. Nathan picked me up and helped me get in his car. Although we were surrounded by police officers, he rushed me to the nearest station, where I filed a report, and they issued a warrant for Raymond.

My right eye was black and swollen, and the skin around it was distorted with one huge knot. Back at the academy on Monday, people stared at me, then said my name as if it were a question. "La Vita?" Some classmates asked what had happened and others, women who recognized the wounds of abuse, simply clicked their tongues and whispered, "Oh girl."

A week later I attended my academy graduation ceremony with liquid makeup caked on my face. For the second time I was at a graduation where I was pleased with my achievements yet sad about the rest of my chaotic life. On this occasion I even captured a piece of history by winning the academy's physical fitness award. People were shocked that a short, petite woman had beat men in running and push-ups. They gave me a rousing standing ovation, and their appreciation boosted the possibilities I saw before me. Wow, I could probably be the first woman on the SWAT team if I want, I thought.

There wasn't an ounce of fat on me. I never ate three meals a day, and I followed a disciplined routine of exercising, running, and doing push-ups. Because of this I fasted only periodically. But inside myself I held disappointment and self-hatred.

After graduation, I followed up on the charges I had filed against Raymond. For evidence, I had pictures taken of me the day after the incident. But when I saw the photos, I was too ashamed to have anyone look at them, so I tore them up.

Raymond called and begged me to meet with him. It is still hard to explain, but whenever I heard his voice, my anger softened and my heart opened. So I agreed to meet him.

This time he was not cocky and arrogant. He was childlike and scared. He cried and begged for forgiveness. He spoke between whimpering. "I didn't mean to hit you, La Vita. But I love you so much, and when I saw you with another man . . . it . . . made . . . me . . . feel . . . crazy.

"Will you drop the charges? I swear, La Vita, I will never touch you again."

In retrospect, his pleas were trite. But at the time I was thinking, This man must be sincere, La Vita, because he's crying.

Men didn't cry. I had never seen my dad or my brother cry. Raymond's tears were proof of his sorrow and love. So I went with him to turn himself in, and I decided to not follow through with the charges.

We started dating each other again. But the calm didn't last long. He simply could not control his rage.

"It's not working, and I don't think it ever will," I told him one day, weary from the jealousy and arguments.

As a police officer, I made things right for people. Yet it seemed I couldn't make things right in my own life.

Chapter Three

Now I wanted to focus on being a good mother and a good police officer. As a single parent, it was challenging to keep up with shift changes at work, which meant making new arrangements with babysitters. Being sick didn't help the situation.

For several weeks I had experienced bad stomach pains, and I wondered if I had developed an ulcer because of the stress in my life. I made an appointment with an internist.

"Before you take the test for an ulcer, I have to give you a pregnancy test. It's standard procedure," he said.

I wasn't concerned. I took the test, then called back for the results so I could set up the appointment for the ulcer test.

I identified myself and held on while the nurse looked up my pregnancy test.

"That test is positive," she said.

"No. I'm calling for the results of the test for La V-i-t-a W-e-a-v-e-r," I said, speaking slowly.

"That test is positive," she repeated.

"That's impossible," I said.

I hung up and called back, figuring she misunderstood me.

"Didn't I tell you it was positive!" the nurse snapped.

I felt like a zombie. Operating on automatic, I dialed Raymond's number. In a solemn, barely audible voice I told him I was pregnant.

He was jubilant. "That's wonderful," he said.

I was in shock. Everything was too familiar: the numbing astonishment, the sick depression that cut to the bone.

It was only later, when it didn't matter, that I discovered that the antibiotics I was taking for bronchitis had reduced the effectiveness of my birth control pills.

I told my older sister I was expecting. She burst into tears. I wasn't surprised.

"Oh my God! You can't be!" she shouted over and over.

After I saw her reaction, I definitely couldn't tell my mother. So I remained silent, practicing in my head the words I would say when the day came that I was forced to tell her. But before that day arrived, I walked into my mother's house one morning and it was clear to me that she knew already. Her face was puffy and her eyes were red and swollen. She looked at me and shook her head as if in disgust. There was only one person cruel enough to tell my mother about the pregnancy before I did. Raymond had found yet another way to express his vengeance.

To say my mother was devastated is putting it mildly. Neither one of us fit well into the other's dreams. A wedge formed between us, and for years we were uncomfortable in each other's presence.

Later, when I turned my life around and my mother saw hope for me, we discussed our misunderstandings.

"I was very, very disappointed in you," she said. "Of all the kids, I knew you would be extremely successful. You had the potential to be not just smart but great."

She thought I intentionally got pregnant because I was mad at her for leaving my father, or for not being there as often as I wanted her. I admitted that at one point I *did* blame her for separating from my father. But that was when I was a kid and needed someone to blame.

"I didn't make those mistakes to spite you," I said.

On some level I sensed that my searching for love was related to my father and my brother Lawrence. Both had been my loving mentors and confidants, and then suddenly they were gone. Something had been missing in my life for a long time and I didn't know how to replace it.

After my mother and I discussed it, we grew closer until we were like sisters, best friends, and mother and daughter all wrapped up in one.

With this pregnancy, my weight zoomed back up. I gained fifty-five pounds. The entire pregnancy was stressful. In nine months I never had one moment of peace. I tried reconciling with Raymond. Looking back, I know I did it because I wanted to silence the whispers and soften the glares I got from people who knew me and who I believed judged me.

To lessen the stress and give myself some joy, I snacked throughout the day on chips and cookies or whatever other junk food was available. I began having anxiety attacks, which sometimes came on in the middle of an argument. I was consumed by fear. My heart pounded so hard and fast I thought I was having a heart attack. The walls of the room drew in closer until it seemed I was standing in a small closet. Everything turned dark.

Food was the only thing that stopped the attacks, or at least stalled them. When an attack hit me suddenly, I gorged myself with whatever food I could grab. The sugar-laden treats satisfied me and calmed me, but the fix was only temporary.

Because I was enduring so much stress and having frequent, painful contractions, the doctor decided to perform a Cesarean early. I went into the hospital on November 21. I was relieved to see the anesthesiologist, as I looked forward to escaping my life while under the influence of medication. But before the anesthesiologist was able to inject me, I started having convulsions. My eyes moved quickly back and forth. My body rippled with uncontrollable muscular contractions. I flung my arms like a rag doll.

The doctors and nurses hurried around, trying to find out what was wrong with me.

"Ms. Weaver! Ms. Weaver!" I heard someone call, but I could not respond. Then the voices faded and a calm came over my body and darkness covered my mind.

I was falling into a black tunnel of depression. I saw it coming for me and I happily gave in to it, traveling deeper. My mind was leaving me and I was relieved. I thought I could reach the end of the tunnel and relax. Until I realized there was no end, that I was traveling, downward, deeper and deeper, spiraling into what seemed to be a bottomless pit.

It was then that I saw the faces of my children, first LaTicia, and then LaTrina. I thought about the baby I was about to give birth to. I remembered the Scriptures I learned when I was growing up, when I read Matthew over and over. I could see the verses of the Bible in red letters.

"Jesus, help me. Don't let me lose my mind," I prayed. "Please, Lord, let me stay for my children."

I saw a flicker of light. Then a blurred image. It was Christ. I knew it was Him.

"Please let me stay," I said.

Chapter Four

I opened my eyes and saw a nurse standing over me.

"Do you know what just happened to you?" she asked.

I wanted to speak, but I couldn't. Although I was coming back from the convulsions, I was still far away. Before I could put together the words to answer her, I was being rushed down the hall and into the delivery room. My sister La Vinia was waiting. I grabbed her hand and squeezed it each time the pain was unbearable. At some point I gave in to the anesthesia.

A nurse's announcement woke me. "You have a new baby girl."

I looked at the small, red baby and felt blessed—even astounded—that I had made it through the pregnancy and delivery. For a brief while I was overwhelmed with joy. Then slowly my mind turned away from the baby and back to everything else I faced. The dark cloud crept up over me again. I sat on the side of my bed and stared into space. I didn't want to eat. I didn't want to talk. "What have I done with my life?" I asked myself over and over.

I had stopped seeing Raymond because I found that the violence in him unleashed violence in me. But one day I let him into my house, thinking that I could show him that we could be friends to each other.

Before long we were rolling on the floor, fighting. The girls called my mother on the phone, screaming. My mother cried hysterically on the other end. After that, I let Raymond see his daughter but I never let him come in the house again. He resented that and once beat my door until he broke the locks.

I went to the police to file charges. Until then, I had kept my life separate from my job, too ashamed to let anyone know what I was going through. But once I filed the charges, someone told my brother, who called me immediately.

Lawrence, a member of the department's renowned SWAT team, was furious. "Tell Raymond if he doesn't remove himself from your life, I will have to remove him," he said.

I delivered the message and Raymond said, "No La Vita, no LaTia." If he couldn't see me, he didn't want to see his daughter either. And he kept his word, because after that he never tried to see LaTia, and he didn't give me any child support for her.

Eventually, I couldn't deal with the constantly changing shifts at the police department. I quit the job because I didn't have sufficient day care. I was a single mother with three children—a baby, a seven-year-old, and a six-year-old.

I felt as though the light at the end of the tunnel was being snuffed out.

I was also dealing once again with weight gain. I had gone from a size 5 before the pregnancy to a size 14 now. Although I wanted to lose weight, food comforted me. So I repeated the cycle of dieting then overeating. My weight constantly fluctuated.

I considered going to a psychiatrist. My sister LaReese suggested God instead. So one afternoon I got on my knees and prayed.

God, I've messed up again. Please open the door for me to go to school again. Show me how to attract the right man, not the vio-

lent, obsessive type but a kind, considerate, loving man who loves me. Forgive me for my mistakes, and give me the strength and courage to make a new life for my children and me—one that honors you. Open me up to your blessings. Amen.

I knew I couldn't wait for God to hand all of this to me. I had to do something to help myself. I had about eight thousand dollars in my savings account, so I enrolled at a local community college, majoring in biological sciences. I also took an aerobics class twice a week. It was uplifting, fun, and exciting, plus I lost a lot of weight—quickly. The movements reminded me of dancing, which I loved.

"Have you ever thought of teaching aerobics?" my instructor asked me one day.

I was surprised. "No," I said.

But my enthusiasm for the exercises was obvious. So the teacher continued to ask me about teaching. At her encouragement I started training at a fitness center. In addition to learning exercises, I studied anatomy and physiology. Eventually, what I thought was just a hobby became an avocation, and I took tests to become an instructor certified by the Aerobics and Fitness Association of America. At school I was taking nutritional courses and learning more about the human body and how to care for it. My plan was to continue my studies at a medical school and become a physician's assistant.

Back in school I did well academically, making the honor roll each semester. I started dating a teacher at the school, a gentle, supportive man who was kind to the girls and me.

With all the changes in my life, I should have been happy, but I wasn't. I started the bingeing cycle all over again. This time I knew how to eat healthy because I had studied nutrition, so I ate healthy during the day and in public, but I binged when I was alone, eating sweets and junk food, things like cake, pies, cookies, and ice cream.

I just couldn't wait to be alone so I could "O.D." on junk food. I was looking better because I was a fitness instructor teaching aerobics regularly. Now I knew how to take care of my body, yet I had a hard time applying the nutritional knowledge because I couldn't gain control of my emotions. Each night after Mark, my new boyfriend, left and I put the kids to bed, I ate chocolate cupcakes, large bags of chips, popcorn drenched in butter and loaded with salt. I needed food that had salt, sugar, and fat because that was the food I could really taste.

There were some occasions when Mark wanted us to spend so much time together that I had trouble breaking away to get my fix. He was a bodybuilder, so I always ate healthy when I was with him. Together, we ate dinners of salmon, rice, and broccoli; baked chicken with baked potatoes and mixed vegetables. But some nights after eating a healthy meal with him, I stopped at Pizza Hut to order a pizza. It was as though I was cheating on him, having a secret affair with food. Not only did I crave sweets, but I also wanted foods laden with fat because they were also the tastiest foods to me. Tasting these foods made me feel alive. Without them, I felt numb.

When I couldn't get away from Mark to eat, I got irritable. My mind felt like it would explode. He knew something was wrong with me, but I couldn't tell him what it was, so he misinterpreted my attitude and took it personally.

I didn't want to hurt him, but I needed my alone time. In my solitude, I ate until I was intoxicated by the overdose of calories. I ate until I threw up or fell into a deep sleep. Then the cycle, which I could not control, started all over again.

I took three psychology courses over two semesters, trying to evaluate and treat myself.

My sister told me again: "La Vita, you need to get into the word of God." True healing could only take place through the word of God, LaReese insisted.

"God, please take away this feeling of hopelessness!" I prayed. "God, help me not hate living!" I sobbed as I drove. I screamed at God and cried. When I was exhausted, a calm washed over me and a silence overwhelmed me.

One thought possessed my mind at that moment: "I have nothing to lose and everything to gain by trying it God's way."

I canceled my appointment with the psychiatrist and immediately started reading the Bible. I read it every day. The more I read, the more I wanted to read. The more I read, the calmer my spirit became. I had less desire to binge and overeat. The words of God filled a void in my inner being.

My sister and I called each other daily to share our feelings about what we had read in the Bible that day.

We were like two little girls with a new toy to share. Then one Sunday, LaReese's sister-in-law invited us to Galilee Baptist Church in Suitland, Maryland, to hear the church's pastor, Rev. Dr. Eugene Weathers. I was transfixed because the very words I read in the Bible were brought to life by his passionate teaching. I left that service even more determined to search the Scriptures and learn more.

Early one morning I came across a Scripture that touched every part of my being. It was Philippians, Chapter 4, verse 13: *"I can do all things through Christ who strengthens me."*

That verse lifted every burden, problem, and fear from my heart.

Then I read Matthew, Chapter 19, verse 26: *"With men this is impossible, but with God all things are possible."*

I pondered its meaning. When I considered my life and what looked important to me, I appeared to be a failure. But if I put all my faith, hope, and trust in God, I was no longer a failure, and the future was full of possibilities.

The knowledge I received from my reading made me see everything differently. This meant I also saw my relationship with my boyfriend in a different way—and this caused problems. It was 1991 and I was entering my third year of college, attending classes part-time. Mark remained a great support to the children and me.

However, the closer I got to God, the further I went from Mark. I felt so overjoyed by the healing taking place in my life that I wanted to give God all of me. I wanted to live the way He wanted me to live. This made dating a struggle, for both Mark and me.

Gradually, the intimate part of our relationship diminished. I avoided him so that I could skirt the possibility of sex. I wanted to live completely for God. Mark did not understand why God would disap-prove of a sexual relationship between two people who loved each other. However, eventually I became completely celibate. I made a decision that I was going to live wholeheartedly for God so that my children and I could experience His abundant blessings. I knew that neither my money, education, job, nor boyfriend could help me when I almost lost my mind or lived with anxiety attacks and overeating be-yond control. No one could help me but God.

Marriage was not the answer for Mark and me because my rela-tionship with God drove us further apart rather than closer together. He believed I was going just a little too far with this God thing.

Although my relationship with Mark was not going well, the kids and I were enjoying time with the other important man in my life: my daddy. He had been sober for ten years by then and had also accepted Christ as Savior. It was like old times. At family get-togethers Daddy was the life of the party again, keeping us in tears from laughing so hard at his stories. But we noticed that he got tired easily and usually left the party early.

"Daddy, why are you limping?" my brother asked one day.

"I have a pain in my right leg sometimes," he said, promising to go to the doctor soon.

At the next family affair I paid closer attention to him—and he was still limping.

"Daddy, did you go check on your leg?" I asked.

"I haven't had time," he said.

When he finally went, the news was bad. He told us they found a spot on his lungs.

"Okay, so what does that mean?" LaReese asked.

He answered as if he were talking about the sun coming up every day. "They say I got cancer," he said.

No one spoke. In my wildest nightmare I had not imagined that my father could be limping because he had cancer. Although he had smoked cigarettes as long as I could remember, he was too full of life and humor to have cancer.

Yet the fact was he had cancer.

The two most important men in my life are leaving me, I thought. Mark and I were not going to make it beyond my celibacy. But the pain over losing him was secondary to the anguish I was experiencing because of my father's illness. And yet I knew I was never truly alone now because I always felt the presence of God. I stayed rooted in the word of God and this sustained me.

Daddy's health deteriorated fast. First, he could no longer walk. Shortly after that, he started wearing diapers. Finally, he was hospitalized. But even while on his back with tubes in his arms, he joked with the doctors and nurses.

When he was under heavy sedation most of the time and unable to talk or hear us, we prayed aloud at his bedside.

"I don't want to die and ruin your holidays," he said repeatedly throughout November.

Thanksgiving passed. In December, he was still concerned about ruining our holidays.

Christmas came and he was heavily sedated. He woke up one morning to find me in the room. "What date is it?" he asked.

"January first," I said.

He smiled and I heard him sigh with relief. I stayed home to get some rest the next day. Of course, that was the day Daddy died. He had survived the holidays. It was January 2, 1992.

The grief was all-consuming and omnipresent. I was happy to have my schoolwork to study, though it was hard to concentrate. When Daddy was sick I told him I was thinking of quitting school. He made me promise to keep going.

My father was dead—and Mark was no longer around to comfort me. I was in anguish. I was learning how to take care of my body by eating right, exercising, and dealing with the root issues of my overeating, which were emotions. I was an emotional eater. To avoid feeling, some people take a drink or a pill; I ate. Whenever I felt negative emotions—anger, pain, regret, or anxiety—food was my "drug" of choice.

I put together a step-by-step health plan based on the Scriptures and on what I had learned about the human body. Still, I sometimes thought God was testing me to see if I would return to my old, unhealthy ways of handling stress rather than relying on Him.

My knees began to ache so much I had to stop teaching aerobics and have surgery on one of my legs. Every time I considered teaching again, that leg hurt. But when I was home dancing to gospel music I was fine. It was strange.

One morning I read a Bible verse I had read many times before, but for some reason on this day it seemed to come to life. It was I Corinthians, Chapter 6, verses 19 and 20: *"Or do you know that your body is the temple of the Holy Spirit who is in you, whom you have from God, and you are not your own? For you were brought at a price; therefore glorify God in your body and in your spirit, which are God's."*

Now I was certain: God wanted me to use my body for His glory.

The most definite sign of what I was to do came when I was exercising. As soon as I did a step, a Scripture came to mind. I repeated the Scripture and the movements fell in sync with the words. I was marching, stepping, and turning to the rhythm of the words of God! It was crazy, but it happened again and again. I didn't try to make up words or fit steps to verses. Everything just popped into my head without effort. I said the Scripture and my body knew exactly what steps to do. Before I knew it, I was working on what I called Hallelujah! Aerobics.

I still find it amazing that when you start walking for God, He will walk you in the direction He wants you to walk in. It's just a matter of surrendering and putting Him first. In the den of my home, God led me in the creation of an exercise program and placed it in my heart to call it Hallelujah! Aerobics for Body and Spirit.

I was so excited that I had to tell someone.

I called my sister LaReese and my mother and told them.

"Every time I move and try to do aerobics to gospel music, Scriptures come into my mind," I said. "It's not all clear to me, but something is happening. I feel God is giving me something."

They believed me because both of them have faith in God and knew that it was possible indeed that God was giving me a new mission. I went over to my mother's house to demonstrate to them.

I repeated one of my favorite verses: *"I can do all things through Jesus Christ who strengthens me."* I gave the verse a rhythm and with each word came a movement and step.

My sister jumped up. "God is leading you!" she said, hugging me.

I copyrighted my routines and the trademark name Hallelujah! Aerobics. Since *hallelujah* means "giving God the highest praise," I called the movements "praise steps." I was giving God praise through aerobics.

During one of my quiet, prayerful periods, God placed it in my heart to do a video of Hallelujah! Aerobics. I know I didn't think of this on my own because I didn't know anything about television production. But I persevered, remembering the Scripture *"With God all things are possible."*

I called a number of television producers to ask for assistance, but since I was not someone with a recognizable name, everyone refused to work with me. Still I heard: *"With God all things are possible."*

So I decided to produce my own video. But first I had to learn how.

I found courses to take at Montgomery College, where I was already a student, and at our local community cable television station. I became a volunteer at both the school's station and at the cable station.

Sometimes I couldn't believe I was taking a path so totally different from that of medicine, the career I had dreamed of for much of my life. I had to be still so I could get clear directions and sort out what I was being told from what I was thinking. I had never been through this before and I didn't understand what I was feeling. Is that you, God? I kept asking. Are *you* telling me to do this?

I now know that God speaks clearly to us in a soft voice. I was expecting lightning, a booming voice, something dramatic. But the soft voice spoke. Yet when I listened, it was clearer than my own thoughts. That voice was whispering, "Television. Television."

"What about medicine?" I asked, doubting.

"Television," came the answer, so clear there was no room for doubt.

I stepped out on faith by first telling several people that I believed I was being called to work in television. Immediately the naysayers were everywhere, each offering a reason why I would fail. Very few people understood, so I stopped telling them. I just moved forward with my plans.

I needed music for the video, so I figured I had to find out about music production. I asked around about musicians and eventually found some who were interested in working with me. Next, I searched for a studio, a crew, and music technicians.

I heard my mantra in my ear: *"With God all things are possible."*

I met a man in the waiting room of my doctor's office, where I was spending a lot of time due to the pain in my knees. I was reading the Bible and writing down aerobics steps. He asked what I was doing and

I explained my project. He told me he was a musician. Out of that chance meeting a collaboration was born, and that musician did the music on my first video.

I heard music in my head, but I didn't know how to write music. So I hummed the melody and stamped out the beat with my feet, and my collaborator wrote down the score.

To save money I gave up my four-bedroom townhouse and moved into the basement of the house where I grew up, sharing it with my sister La Vinia and her two boys. This was a major adjustment for my girls and me, but I was having major financial difficulties. I was receiving almost no child support from either father. Meanwhile, I had to go the doctor frequently—at $120 a visit—because of my knees, and I had no health insurance. By working for a temp agency and taking personal clients whenever I could, I put aside any extra pennies to save for the video production.

I really didn't see how the film was going to be financed and finished, but I believed that if God said it, that settled it. One day I was on my knees praying when I heard that quiet still voice tell me that someone would give me the additional funds to complete the project. Before I could get up off my knees, the phone rang and my mother was on the other end.

"La Vita," she said. "I know that God is leading you to do something great with your life. So I'm going to do whatever is necessary to give you the money you need to complete the video."

I thanked my mother, but I also shouted my thanks to God. He had come through on His word again.

Making a video was not cheap. I had to pay for everything—my own training, studio time, musicians, tapes, packaging, graphics, artwork, and any small thing that came up. Of course, I needed people to exercise in the videotape, so I used some ladies from my church. They were regular people like those who I imagined would watch the tapes—different shapes, complexions, heights, and sizes.

We practiced in my basement, pushing back the furniture. My participants wore T-shirts and leotards, but nothing fancy. The focus was not on the body; it was on health.

The next step was packaging. I got assistance in creating a cover design. The day I completed the first package with a video inside, I drove to my church and ran inside with it, screaming, "Pastor! Pastor! It's done!"

Before long, the word spread and people called me to order copies. I submitted the tape for consideration to a main resource guide for people in the fitness business. I didn't think it would make it since it was a Christian tape with the mention of Jesus throughout it. But to my surprise the tape was chosen.

Meanwhile, I was working as a personal trainer, wearing a size 5, and weighing about 125 pounds. When I told people I used to weigh 200 pounds, they didn't believe me. They thought I couldn't relate to their challenges with food and health. But I took an old photo of myself to one of my classes, and people started treating me differently because now they knew I understood them.

I sent a "before" and "after" photo of myself to *Heart and Soul* magazine, and someone from the magazine called to say they wanted to profile me. During that interview I talked about my addiction to food for the first time. Around the same time, people also started asking me to do workshops, and I began the Fit for God workshops, developing a fitness program based on the steps I had used in my own weight management.

Then two other magazines, *Shape* and *Excellence,* published my story. "Okay, God, if this is what you want me to do, I will do it," I said.

I created three additional videos. In addition to offering them through the mail, I put them in Christian bookstores in my area.

I went to a church one day to give a workshop, but the hall where we were to meet wasn't available. I was going to leave, but people asked me to speak in the sanctuary instead. I was hesitant but I wanted to satisfy them, so I went to the car and got my Bible. As I stood to speak, the words just came.

From that day forth I have been giving public speeches as well as conducting my fitness programs. Now I follow whatever God asks me to do. I was led into the ministry training program at church. I speak at women's retreats, health fairs, political conferences for women— wherever I am called.

But God's plan for me is still unfolding. I was watching Kenneth Copeland on Trinity Broadcasting Network and saw a testimony by a woman who had started a program for kids, operating on faith. I knew I possessed that same kind of faith and decided to use it. I sent a video of my story to *The 700 Club* and to Trinity Broadcasting Network.

The 700 Club contacted me first. They interviewed me and ran a depiction of my story on their program. After receiving a tremendous response from the airing of the story, they repeated the show several times.

A year passed and I forgot about the video sent to TBN. But I was watching a show on the network one day when this deep, intense feeling came over me. I *knew* I was going on TBN, and this truth touched my soul and made me cry.

"What's wrong, Mommy?" one of my daughters asked.

"I'm going on TBN," I said, tears streaming down my cheeks.

A week later a man from TBN called me.

"You're playing a joke on me, right?" I managed to say.

But it was not a joke. The man said Lee Haney, eight-time Mr. Olympia, was putting together a Christian fitness show called *TotaLee Fit* and needed a cohost. I knew this had to be part of God's divine plan, because at the time I was producing a show called *Eternally Fit,* a Christian fitness show aired on my local cable station.

The man calling from TBN said that somehow the owners of the TBN network, Paul and Jan Crouch, ended up with my tape.

"They think you and Lee Haney will be a great couple because of your personalities," he said.

The network regularly receives hundreds of tapes from all over the country, and generally staff members screen them. No one could explain how the owners had wound up with my tape. But it was no mystery to me. As far as I was concerned, God directed the circumstances.

Next, I was also invited to give my testimony on the popular TBN show *Praise the Lord*. I was nervous because God was taking me out of my comfort zone. A private person, I would now share my problems of overeating and depression with people around the world. But again I prayed, and on the show when I opened my mouth, the words flowed.

The response was incredible. Women from all over the country wrote me to say how much my testimony helped them.

As the mail piled up, God placed it in my heart that I could reach more people if I wrote a book. So even though I didn't know anything about writing a book, I began writing notes and an outline.

That was all I had to do—to act on faith—for God to make a way. Denise Stinson, a literary agent, saw a magazine article on me and called.

"You should consider writing a book," she said. "I'd be happy to represent you."

Of course I was excited, but I hesitated enough to say, "Let me pray on it first."

I wanted to make sure Denise was the right person, and I wanted to make sure I was moving in the direction God wanted me to go.

I know that this book is just another step, a piece of the journey God continues to reveal to me. More than anything else, I want to share with my readers what I know to be true: The Spirit of God is real.

The
Eight-Week
Fit for God
Program

Week One

Have a Positive Attitude

Then God Said, Let There Be Light; and There Was Light.
—Genesis 1:3

I f you are tired of struggling with how to lose weight and want to create a complete, new you, you can learn from God, the "Master Creator." Fit for God is based on God's word found in the Bible. In Hosea 4:6, the Lord says, *"My people are destroyed from lack of knowledge."*

In other words, what you don't know can actually kill you. Not knowing that eating a diet high in cholesterol and saturated fat can cause a buildup of plaque on the walls of your arteries and lead to a fatal heart attack. Not knowing all the wonderful benefits of exercise for disease prevention can lead to serious illness and even death.

But before you take the first step toward better health, you must have faith. In Week One, you receive tips for boosting your faith and holding on to it. You will write affirmations in your journal, read Bible verses, and repeat a prayer to help you create a positive attitude and prepare you for the challenge that follows. What you think and the words you speak to yourself will determine whether or not you can maintain healthy habits once you learn them. Always remember: You are not in this battle alone. God, our Father, walks beside you.

You may have forgotten the power He has bestowed upon you. Because you are created in the image of God, you too have the power to speak things into existence just as God did when He created the universe. But He didn't do it overnight.

Genesis 1:3–5 says, *"Then God said, 'Let there be light,' and there was light. And God saw the light, that it was good; and God divided the light from the darkness. God called the light Day, and the darkness He called Night. So the evening and the morning were the first day"* (NKJV).

Think about it. The omnipotent Almighty God, who is Maker and Supreme Ruler over heaven and earth, had the power to do everything at once. But as awesome as He is, as magnificent as His divine power and glory is, God devised a step-by-step plan for creation of the universe. This plan was the preparation for His ultimate creation. He had to put some things in place to prepare for His "master creation."

Of everything that exists in the universe, do you know what His "master creation" was? It was you and me. He wanted us to be complete and have everything we needed, so He didn't do a rush job. He had to make sure we had the right atmosphere to inhale oxygen so we could breathe. He had to make sure we had water to drink, dry ground to stand on, light to see, food to eat, and the sun to sustain life. Before He made humankind, there was a preparation process so that His creation would live and not die.

In Ephesians 5:1, it states, *"Be imitators of God."* If you want permanent success in weight loss—I'm talking about a lasting lifestyle change, not losing weight one month and putting it back on the following month—follow the steps of God, the greatest planner.

God didn't do anything haphazardly. Even when He gave Joshua the plan to conquer the Promised Land, He didn't tell him to overtake it all at once. He had Joshua and his followers march into the land of Canaan and then divide the territories they were to conquer.

They conquered it in sections until finally they overtook the entire land. This strategic plan was so successful that officers in modern-day war have been known to study the strategy Joshua used.

I want you to view your weight management plan the same way. Don't read these steps and immediately try to do them all at once. If you do, you'll set yourself up for failure and disappointment. Permanent weight loss involves gradual change. Work on one step at a time until you have conquered that particular area, then move on to new territory.

I simply cannot overemphasize how important this is. Please take this advice seriously. Don't frustrate yourself by trying to master each step of the Fit for God program immediately. Learn bit by bit. You can try to conquer each area in the order it is presented in the book, or you can pick them in an order you believe will make them easier for you. I've discovered that every individual is different.

Remember that improvement is what you're striving for. So don't beat yourself up if you feel you have not perfected a particular step. Eventually, you can come back and reexamine the difficult step.

The very first line of the Bible starts with God creating the heavens and the earth. The next verse describes the condition of the earth before God gave order to the universe. It states that the earth was void and without form and filled with darkness. Can you relate that to the way you may feel about your body at times?

I didn't like the shape of my body when I gained a lot of weight. The only shape I had was round. I remember looking in the mirror and seeing that my twenty-four-inch waistline had been transformed into a tire rim. This shape had me feeling depressed and unhappy about my image and myself. That was a very dark period in my life.

In the beginning, the earth was in a similar state, but God still created something beautiful with what He had. Although God saw that the earth was in a chaotic state of disorder and confusion, He still proceeded with His plan. Although He saw the earth as formless matter, He didn't focus on its present state. God must have felt hopeful and positive about the beautiful change that would take place. He didn't focus on what the earth was at that time; He focused on what it would be.

So in Week One, focus on "the light": Have a positive attitude.

When you're struggling with all the issues that will arise in this battle, have faith. When you look in the mirror and don't like what you see, know by faith that you will change. What is faith? Faith is having trust, confidence, or belief in someone or something. For instance, many of us may have faith in our paychecks or jobs paying our bills. We may have faith in a promotion getting us a new house or car. We may have faith in our cars getting us from one place to another. We even place our faith in loved ones, coworkers, or friends.

But Mark 11:22 says, *"Have faith in God."* Just think about it— without God none of these people or things would even exist.

Hebrews 11:1 says, *"Now faith is the substance of things hoped for, the evidence of things unseen."* Let's examine this for a moment. It says faith is what I don't see, but it is the evidence of what I hope for. If you can see it, you don't need faith. What you need to hope for is in God's power and His word. Verse 3 continues to say that by faith we believe the worlds were created by God's spoken word. So we believe that God created the earth, even though we didn't see Him do it. The Bible says it; therefore, we believe . . . That's faith.

When you don't like what the scale reads, or if you feel uncomfortable in your clothes, have a positive attitude. Remember that God is standing with you, and where there is God, there is hope. Know that with God you can do all things but fail.

Forget trying or wanting to look like someone else. Everyone is different. We have different shapes, heights, body types, and so on.

Forget the body images you see on magazines in the food checkout lines and the stars you see on television.

Instead, fill any doubt in your mind with the words of Mark, Chapter 9, verse 23: *"All things are possible to him who believes."*

Anyway, most of the images we see on television and in magazines are not realistic. For instance, the average female model is about 5´8˝–5´10˝ and a size 4. In reality the average woman is about 5´5˝ and a size 10.

You want to strive to be healthy. And if being healthy is a size 10 for you, that's fine. Instead of looking at a picture of someone else in a magazine, find an old photo of yourself at a desired weight and use that as your guide. Put it in a prominent place where you see it often. If you don't have such a photo, use your imagination. See yourself the way you want to be.

Be careful with this exercise. You must be realistic. My desire for years was to have the body I had as a teenager, which only frustrated me because that was not a realistic goal. After years of disappointment, I finally got real with myself. When I had that old body I was a lot younger and didn't have three children. I had to learn how to work with who I am today.

Be positive. If God could work with what He had—a dark, void, chaotic state of matter—and create a beautiful, vast universe filled with galaxies and planets and arrayed with stars of various shapes and sizes, you can work with what you have to create the best you can be. Even if your past experiences have left you feeling it's impossible to lose weight, remember that this time you won't be alone. The basis of the Fit for God plan is to understand and acknowledge that the Almighty God, who is the sovereign Lord of the universe, is right there to help you.

The Bible says if you acknowledge God in all your ways, He will direct your path. So trust God as He directs you every step of the way. With God, nothing is impossible.

According to Genesis 1:3, God spoke in the positive. He said, *"Let there be light,"* and the Bible says light appeared. Consider how powerful that is. God spoke the light into existence. *You* also have the power to speak into existence the results you desire. Well, that starts right here, with the power in *your* mouth. If you've been using your mouth to put the weight on, now it's time to start using your mouth to take the weight off.

The Bible not only shows us what God expects from His children, but it clearly demonstrates how we can overcome various challenges. One of my favorite descriptions of the holy book is B-I-B-L-E = Basic Instructions Before Leaving Earth.

Check out some of these instructions for your mouth:

Proverbs 18:21: *"Death and life are in the power of the tongue, and those who love it will eat its fruit."* This means we can speak life and death into our very situations. We can speak defeat or victory. Because whatever we speak will be our fruit.

Proverbs 16:24: *"Pleasant words are a honeycomb, sweetness to the soul and healing to the bones."* In other words, if you want good health, start speaking good health. Stop saying, "I can't do it." If you want to overcome the battle of the bulge, start speaking as if you *will* overcome the battle of the bulge. Start speaking words of life, words that are sweet to your soul and health for your body. Speak it, knowing God is there to help you achieve your goal.

In other words, you have the ability to make something happen. This biblical concept is so real that many people, including psychotherapists and psychiatrists, have written books on the power of positive thinking. Motivational speakers use many of the principles found in the Bible to encourage people to strive for success in every area of life.

Just as positive speaking works, so does negativity. Remember, the Bible says life and death are in the power of your tongue. So you have to be careful not to let negative words proceed from your mouth. If you say you're a failure, guess what? You'll be a failure. If you say you can't do it, guess what? You won't do it.

The children of Israel saw God bring them miraculously out of Egypt and divide the Red Sea. They saw Him lead them and protect them through the desert. Yet they constantly complained. When the ten spies said they could not make it to the Promised Land and the people complained and cried, they didn't make it. But Joshua and Caleb, who said they could make it with God, made it.

I can remember speaking negatively about my weight and myself then acting upon what I spoke. I can remember thinking, "I'm fat and I'll never lose this weight." And guess what? I stayed fat and I didn't lose the weight. It seems logical that if I thought I was fat, I would do something about it. But instead if I was disappointed with what I saw when I stepped on a scale, I'd complain and immediately grab a large bag of chips, Cheetos, cookies, cupcakes, ice cream, or all of them at one sitting. My negative attitude and the negative words I spoke from my mouth had the same power as the extra calories I ate.

I didn't begin to see positive results until I developed a more positive attitude and learned how to allow positive words to proceed from my mouth.

This concept also applies to your thoughts, for the Bible says as a man thinketh so is he. Begin to fill your mind with positive thoughts. Before God could actually speak Creation into existence He had to think about it first. Think it, speak it, and watch it come to pass.

Put these thoughts in your mind, and then speak them aloud:

"I will lose weight and keep it off."

"I know I will succeed."

"God is here to help me."

"My body will be fit and healthy."

"I will be set free from my bondage with food and this 'body trap.'"

"I am not a failure."

"I will have control over my eating habits."

"I will be fit for God."

Although you may not feel or even believe what you are saying right away, if you keep on saying it, you will eventually believe it and act upon it. In Mark, Chapter 9, when a father wanted his child healed, Jesus said, *"All things are possible to him who believes."* The Bible then says that the father of the child cried out with tears and said, *"Lord, I believe; help my unbelief!"*

So if you're having trouble fully believing, you can be honest with God and tell Him you need help. As your faith gets stronger, you will automatically begin to take the necessary steps to achieve your healthy new body.

If you don't know what to speak or think, pick up that powerful book we are to live by: the Holy Bible. Try reading these verses to find out what God says about you, then feel your Father's truth in your heart and start speaking into existence the healthy body you desire:

- Philippians 4:13—*"I can do all things through Christ who strengthens me."*
- Psalm 139:14—*". . . I am fearfully and wonderfully made; marvelous are your works, and that my soul knows very well."*

There are many examples of people speaking things into existence. What seemed totally unheard of became possible by a spoken word of faith—and divine intervention. In the Book of Ezekiel, Chapter 37, Ezekiel spoke life into dead, dry bones, which represented the Jews who were in bondage. Those dead bones came to life, stood up on their feet, and became an exceedingly great army. With the power of your tongue and the help of God, you can also speak exceedingly great things into your life.

I still remember a woman named Sylvia who attended a Fit for God workshop and was very serious about the program. One day in class she shared with everyone the steps of the plan that she had successfully incorporated into her life. She included all of the steps except the step from Week One. When I asked her about this first step, she said she struggled with it more than the others.

"I can always say something positive about others, but I don't have anything positive to say about myself," she said. "I'm in the class only because I know God wants me to be healthy."

"What do you expect to gain from the class?" I asked.

She answered, "I want to live healthy so I can be what God wants me to be."

"That's a good start," I told her. "Your positive statement is: 'I will live healthier so I can be what God wants me to be.'"

If, like Sylvia, you find it hard to speak positively about yourself, think about why you are reading this book and what goals you want to obtain.

The best way to keep a positive attitude is to say something positive about yourself every day. I'm not talking about words of vanity, but words of encouragement as you give God the glory for what He is going to do in your life. Look in the mirror and say, "I am a child of God, perfect in every way." In the shower, repeat: "Each day I gain more knowledge to make my body fit." As you put on your shoes, say, "You guide my feet and my ways. Victory is mine."

Have fun. Speak the words to an imaginary beat. Dance to the words; pick one phrase and walk in rhythm to it throughout the day.

The Book of Philippians was written by the apostle Paul, who was in prison awaiting trial and possible execution for preaching the gospel of Jesus Christ. Still, he used the words "joy" and "rejoice" numerous times in his writing.

What was Paul's secret to his joy? It was his focus. He didn't focus on his present circumstances. He focused on Jesus Christ, who was the center of his life, and how joyous it was to be a child of God. In Philippians 4:8, he writes: *"Finally, brethren, whatever things are true, whatever things are noble, whatever things are just, whatever things are pure, whatever things are lovely, whatever things are of good report, if there is any virtue and if there is anything praiseworthy, meditate on these things."*

You have to meditate or think on the things that are good and lovely, those things of God. You may have to train yourself to do it by paying attention to your thoughts, then shifting them when you find you are focused on the bad. I know it's difficult to find the positive in the extra fat you see in the mirror. I know it's difficult to focus on the positive when you feel uncomfortable in your clothes and feel everyone is looking at you and judging you.

I vividly remember feeling totally disgusted with my body, with the extra weight, the dimples in my thighs, the roll around my waist, and the bulge in my stomach. I thought the backs of my arms were so flabby they flapped like a bird's wings. I could feel my buttocks shake like Jell-O when I walked fast.

It wasn't easy for me to find anything positive in the beginning. But I made up my mind I was going to change. Change starts in your mind. When a negative thought comes to your mind, don't entertain it. Immediately focus on something positive. If you find it difficult to find the positive, just as I did in the beginning, start by focusing on things we take for granted such as: "I can breathe without an oxygen machine"; "I can walk"; "I have shelter, food to eat, clothes to wear."

After some months of repeating such statements and writing them in my journal, I was able to look outside myself and see the good in the trees, the sky, and the air, and in the other good and beautiful creations of God. Realizing that I was one of God's beautiful creations helped me change my attitude about myself.

As you pay attention to your own thoughts, notice your thoughts about others. Are you frequently criticizing others? In most instances, criticism is a reflection of what the criticizer thinks of herself.

Sarah was a thirty-four-year-old mother who went to a size 15 from a size 10 after she had her children. Whenever Sarah saw a woman who was also overweight, she said, "Oh, she's fatter than me." Or, "Am I that fat?"

I could relate to her. After having been extremely self-critical, I then always saw flaws in others. I encouraged Sarah to deal with the real issue instead of criticizing others. In my own case, as with many people, putting others down made me feel better about myself. But I found the feeling was only temporary. Eventually you have to deal with what you don't like about yourself.

There are others who don't criticize intentionally, but were put down or criticized often during childhood. Now they have the same bad habit.

Learn to replace negative statements—including those about others—with positive statements. Practice until you develop a more positive attitude and the thoughts come naturally. If you're going to succeed in losing weight, your attitude is very important. Your attitude about yourself—and others—can determine whether you succeed or fail.

Sarah was eventually able to understand the root issue of her behavior and, with help, change her attitude. She began to encourage others, which made her feel good and in turn helped motivate her to do something about her own weight.

It was in working on developing my own positive attitude that I realized my problem with food had less to do with what I was eating and more to do with what was eating me. I couldn't move forward, emotionally, to a brighter future because I was busy focusing on all of my regrets from the past. I had health, three beautiful daughters who were great kids and doing well in school, a family, a home, and a future. But I couldn't see my blessings or any type of future because the light was covered by a thick, dark cloud of regrets.

Anxiety, stress, and depression are the reasons I had no control over my food intake. I was an emotional eater. I still am to this very day. So I live this Fit for God program daily and probably will until the day I die. Although I'm healed from my past, when I'm stressed I get a mad craving to eat. I now know how to control it. Now I deal with the issue instead of allowing the issue to grow until it controls me.

The La Vita who appeared confident and strong on the outside was really a nervous wreck who made some terribly foolish decisions. I thought I was doing fine, but when things are inside of you, they will come out one way or another and manifest themselves in other areas of your life. In the past I didn't even talk to my mother or sister, who were the two closest people in my life. I didn't talk to my best girlfriend, either. My hidden issues came out as overeating, bingeing, anxiety attacks, depressions, anger, lack of patience, and eventually a nervous breakdown.

My healing began when I started talking to others about these issues. It was an exhilarating experience. I felt free from years of bondage. When I stopped living a lie and shared my experiences, the truth set me free. I felt as if I had wings and could fly above any and all obstacles. It was the feeling that sparked the idea for the logo of my company: a pair of wings.

It is important to separate the darkness from the light in your life. Exposing the dark issues of hurt, pain, discomfort, or disappointment will eventually allow you to see the light of truth. Many people don't want to accept the truth. They hide it because they don't want to face the hurt, or they feel embarrassed, ashamed, or guilty about what occurred to them.

When you hide painful experiences, they aren't really hidden. They will manifest themselves in other areas of your life. The way they show up varies from person to person. They may come out as anger, bitterness, frustration, stress, constant fatigue, drug use, alcohol abuse, or even overeating.

If you've been struggling with losing weight and have tried various programs and diets, your reason for failure may also be hidden areas of darkness. I've spoken to hundreds of people all around the country, and I can tell you for a fact that many people who have experienced failure in weight management and struggled with overeating year after year have had other underlying culprits contributing to their lack of success in weight management.

Week One is very important because, once I give you the health and fitness knowledge you need for your desired goal, you need to be able to hold on to your results. If you have other underlying issues besides wanting to know how to care for your body, now is the time to deal with them.

Many of us cannot enjoy the brightness in life because we allow the darkness to consume us. So how do you enjoy the light that's already in your life?

Participate in activities that will boost your faith and therefore allow you to develop a positive attitude. And remember: You are not alone.

PRAYER

You can write this prayer on an index card so you can keep it in your pocketbook or suit pocket to read whenever you need a boost, perhaps as you head to a restaurant at lunchtime or before sitting down to dinner.

Dear God,
The Bible says if I acknowledge you in all my ways (in everything I do), you will direct my path (lead me every step of the way). The

*Bible also says that all power in heaven and on earth belongs to
you. Therefore, I am relying on your power to lead me through
every step of this program. I am relying on your power to strengthen
me and help me overcome any and all challenges. I am relying on
your power to give me energy when I just don't feel like doing it. I
am relying on your power to renew my mind, and my taste buds, so
I can make better food choices. I am relying on your power to help
me make healthy lifestyle changes a permanent part of my life, so I
can be all you created me to be. I am going to do what I humanly
can, while relying on your power to do what I can't. I believe according to Your Word that it is possible for me to finally win this
battle of the bulge and get the results I've been long waiting for. I
am now thanking you in advance for your help as I go through the
Fit for God program. In Jesus' name I pray. Amen.*

ACTIVITIES

1. Speak your desires into existence. Look in the mirror each
morning, right into your own eyes, and make a positive statement
such as, "This is temporary, this weight is coming off, and I will be
healthy, fit, energetic, and free. I look forward to my new freedom."

2. Study the Scriptures. Record your Study Scriptures on index
cards so you can carry them with you. Throughout this book I include what I call Study Scriptures that pertain to the topics in each
week of the Fit for God program. Write them in your journal. Repe-
tition will make them become a part of your permanent thinking. Try
Psalm 139:14—". . . *I am fearfully and wonderfully made; marvelous
are your works, and that my soul knows very well.*" And Philippians
4:13—"*I can do all things through Christ who strengthens me.*"

3. Write down the good in your life. Write at least five examples in your journal. Some of my personal examples are: God gave me
three beautiful, healthy daughters; God gave me a beautiful mother, a

fun-loving father, and four loving brothers and sisters; God has always met all of my basic needs such as shelter, food, and clothes, even during times when I really didn't know how I was going to make it; God has given me another opportunity to live healthier. I'm free through Christ Jesus, and one day I'm going to spend eternity with Him.

4. Write down five things you like about yourself. Please include two to three statements about your physical appearance. My personal journal entries when I was overweight included: I like my almond-shaped eyes; I like my smile; I like the love and compassion for others God has given me; I like my attitude of laughter; I have nice feet.

5. Pay attention to your thought pattern. (a) Think about the health goal you want to achieve. (b) Write down the negative thoughts that come to mind. (c) Write down the opposite of the negative thought, or a positive affirmation, five times. Read the affirmation aloud.

Example: Goal—(a) I want to lose weight and tone my body; (b) Negative thought: I'll never lose this weight and get firm; (c) Affirmation: I will lose weight and get firm (repeat five times).

6. Encourage others. Make it your business to compliment others. Tell someone something positive daily or at least twice a week. You don't have to lie or exaggerate. Learn to see the good in others. Many people are always down because they focus on their own problems. Look outside of yourself at others and you will find that everyone has challenges. Watching how people meet those challenges can motivate you.

7. Walk. Walk in your own neighborhood for ten minutes. If you have to, take the dog for a walk, or walk in your favorite mall. Don't stop to look or shop. Many malls have early-morning walking programs before the stores open. When you're ready, join a mall program. If you live near a park you may find people walking there also; or when you're parking to go in a store, don't always choose the space closest to the door; try parking a couple of blocks away or across the lot.

If you have a sit-down job, make it a habit to get up and walk. For example, if you have to use the restroom, use the one farthest down the hall. If you ride the subway, walk up the escalators. If you catch a bus, walk to the stop a little farther down the road. Make walking a part of your daily health routine.

TIP: Memorize your Study Scriptures and repeat them in your mind or aloud while you walk. You'll soon discover that you are walking by faith because faith comes and grows only by the Word of God.

8. Get a journal. It doesn't have to be a fancy book; it can be a spiral notebook. After speaking aloud your positive statement, record it and the date in your journal. Do this each day. You don't have to have a different statement each day. You can repeat the same statement until you feel like saying another one.

Writing in a journal will play an important role in your success. Write to your heart's content. Write down what you eat, how you feel, and the emotions that trigger your overeating. Write down where you are and who you are with when you overeat. Write down the issues you are aware of when you start and those you discover along the way. Write your weekly and monthly goals. Just write to God. Habakkuk 2:2–3 reads, *"Then the Lord answered me and said: Write down the vision and make it plain on tablets, that he may run who reads it. For the vision is yet for an appointed time; but at the end it will speak, and it will not lie. Though it tarries, wait for it; because it will surely come, it will not tarry."*

Habakkuk was a prophet of God who was deeply disturbed about the injustice and darkness he saw in Judah's society. He asked God how long He would allow these conditions to remain among His people. He made a desperate appeal to God, asking Him when things would change. When God answered Habakkuk, instead of telling him when things would change, God told him to write and wait.

Although God wasn't referring to weight loss, this is a biblical principle that we can still use today. I can definitely relate to the importance of writing and waiting or being a "writer in wait." In addition to changing my eating habits and becoming more active, writing was one of the most important things I did to help myself lose weight and win the battle of the bulge. Once I got in the writing habit, there were many times when I was emotionally upset, but instead of grabbing a bag of chips or a box of cookies I grabbed my journal. Instead of allowing my spoon to do the damage by eating a whole pint of ice cream at one sitting, I used my pen to write out my negative emotions. By the time I was finished, my mad craving to overindulge had completely subsided. This was how I discovered the moods or attitudes that affected my intake of food. As I waited for my results, I wrote. This is what God was telling Habakkuk. He told him to write the vision down and be patient. It may seem like it's taking a while, but it will surely come at the "write" time.

While you're waiting for your results, write and be patient. If you lose weight too fast without discovering the reasons why you overeat and learning how to deal with your issues, you'll regain the weight fast. But if you're writing and waiting, you'll discover so much about you and your eating habits. And before you know it, you'll get the results you want and will learn how to keep them. Also remember to keep the faith as you're waiting. Habakkuk 2:4 reads, *"But the just shall live by his faith."* So your faith and trust in God being there will strengthen you as you're waiting for your results. Discover the freedom and victory in writing, and while you're waiting, learn how to enjoy the good in your life. As a matter of fact, write down the good, too.

Create a positive attitude by getting rid of the issues that may be stopping you

The Word of God can help you overcome any obstacle in your life. If you've allowed one of these reasons to stop you from being healthy, read and meditate on the Scripture that relates to your issue.

1. ABUSE

I have spoken to many people who were abused during childhood or later in life by their spouses or their own children. Many emotions accompany abuse—anger, bitterness, guilt, and shame. It's important to seek proper counseling, if needed, and to deal with your feelings as you allow God to heal you through His Word. **Psalm 107:20** *He sent His word and healed them, and delivered them from their destructions.*

2. AGE

You are never too old to be used by God or to get started living healthier. If you exercise regularly and eat healthy, you will feel younger. **Psalm 103:2–5** *Bless the Lord, O my soul, and forget not all His benefits; who forgives all your iniquities, who heals all your diseases, who redeems your life from destruction, who crowns you with loving-kindness and tender mercies, who satisfies your mouth with good things, so that your youth is renewed like the eagle's.*

3. ANGER

Anger is not a sin, but if it's not dealt with in a godly manner it can cause harm to you and others. Some people are too angry with themselves to make a change. Forgive yourself. **Ephesians 4:26–27** *Be angry, and do not sin; do not let the sun go down on your wrath, nor give place to the devil.*

4. ANXIETY

God doesn't want you to be anxious about anything. He wants you to pray, tell Him your concerns, and allow His peace to fill your heart and mind. **Philippians 4:6–7** *Be anxious for nothing, but in everything by prayer and supplication, with thanksgiving, let your requests be made known to God; and the peace of God, which surpasses all understanding, will guard your hearts and minds through Christ Jesus.*

5. ATTENTION

As odd as it may seem, some people want to remain unhealthy because they enjoy the attention and concern they get from others. If you desire to be the center of attention, seek God and He will give you all the attention you need. **II Chronicles 7:14–15** *If My people who are called by My name will humble themselves, and pray and seek My face, and turn from their wicked ways, then I will hear from heaven, and will forgive their sin and heal their land. Now my eyes will be open and my ears attentive to prayer made in this place.*

6. BELITTLEMENT

You may feel you cannot accomplish anything because other people have put you down for so long. But trust who you are in God and know that He specifically created you for a good work. After all, it's His opinion that really matters. **Ephesians 2:10** *For we are His workmanship, created in Christ Jesus for good work, which God prepared beforehand that we should walk in them.*

7. BITTERNESS

Bitterness can eat at you like a canker sore. God tells us to get rid of all bitterness and forgive. **Ephesians 4:31–32** *Let all bitterness, wrath, anger, clamor and evil speaking be put away from you, with all malice. And be kind to one another, tenderhearted, forgiving one another, even as God in Christ forgave you.*

8. BLAME

Take responsibility for your own actions. Don't blame others. If someone doesn't cook for you or go walking with you, that's still no reason for you to neglect your health. Even if others have done something to hurt you, you can't blame them for your overeating. Examine your own actions. God is going to hold you accountable for what you do. **Ezekiel 18:20** *The soul who sins shall die. The son shall not bear the guilt of the father, nor the father bear the guilt of the son. The righteousness of the righteous shall be upon himself, and the wickedness of the wicked shall be upon himself.*

9. DEPRESSION

Many people have experienced depression, even some of the great men and women of God. Remember when the great prophet Elijah was depressed in I Kings, Chapter 19, and he asked God to take his life? The angel of the Lord told him to get up and eat because he needed his strength. He ate, then got up and went to seek a Word from the Lord. When you feel down and out, instead of focusing on your situation, put your hope in God and meditate on the One who can bring you out. **Psalm 71:5** *For you are my hope, O Lord God; you are my trust from my youth.*

10. DISCOURAGEMENT

When it was time for Joshua to conquer the Promised Land, God assured him repeatedly that he didn't have to be discouraged because God was with Him. When things tend to seem too difficult in life, you can rest assured that God is right by your side. **Joshua 1:9** *Have I not commanded you? Be strong and of good courage; do not be afraid or dismayed, for the Lord your God is with you wherever you go.*

Week Two
Drink Plenty of Water

Then God Said, Let the Waters under the Heavens Be
Gathered Together into One Place, and Let the Dry Land
Appear; and It Was So.

—Genesis 1:9

After creating the light, God turned His attention to the waters. *"Let there be a firmament in the midst of the waters, and let it divide the waters from the waters. Thus God made the firmament, and divided the waters which were under the firmament from the waters which were above the firmament; and it was so"* (Genesis 1:6–7). God divided the water by a firmament, which is the sky or heaven. He divided the water in preparation for the "hydrologic cycle" or "water cycle."

Through the "hydrologic cycle" the earth will never run out of water. The water just changes from one state to another, to be used all over again. For example, the heat from the sun causes evaporation from rivers, lakes, seas, and oceans. This water vapor rises, cools, and condenses into tiny droplets that form the clouds we see in the sky.

At various times these droplets in the clouds form rain, hail, or snow. These forms of water return to the earth in a continuous cycle to replenish and restore, and wind currents keep the water moving around the globe.

Water is needed for man and animals to drink. It is needed for vegetation to grow, so animals and man can have food to eat. Water is needed for fish and other animals of the sea to live.

Water is so important for life that we can survive days, weeks, maybe months without food, but only days without water. The human body is about 55 to 70 percent water, and no bodily function takes place without water. But we humans don't have a water cycle like that of the earth.

Water is the most important and most abundant natural resource, yet it is also the one we take for granted the most. If your throat isn't dry and you don't have sweat pouring off your forehead, you tend to take it for granted. But water does a lot more than just satisfy your thirst. Among its duties, it carries nutrients throughout the body, adds moisture to body tissues, softens stool, helps cushion your joints, and aids in the regulation of body temperature. Therefore, the human body continuously loses water throughout the day, and water molecules floating around in the atmosphere cannot be reabsorbed back into the body. We lose water through urination, stool excretion, respiration, sweating, and evaporation from the skin. Consequently, just as God planned a "water cycle" to replenish the water on earth, we need to create a "water cycle" for our bodies by making a conscious effort to ensure an ongoing intake of water.

Water is the sustainer of all life on the earth, just as God is the creator and ultimate sustainer of life on earth. All life forms were made from water; God made all creation.

Water can have a relaxing and calming effect, yet it can be destructive in the form of floods that can uproot trees and sweep cars away. God is so loving and kind, yet His wrath can cause great destruction, such as when He completely destroyed the cities of Sodom and Gomorrah for their disobedience to God. And of all the substances known, water is the only one known to man that, at earth's ordinary temperatures, exists in three states: liquid, solid, and gas; God has three persons: Father, Son, and Holy Spirit.

Water is used symbolically in the Bible. In the Book of John, Chapter 4, Jesus Christ refers to Himself as having *"living water,"* saying that those who drink of the water He has to offer will never thirst again. He's saying that what He has is the major source for life, the major source for satisfying that longing, craving, desire: the thirst in your soul. He continues to say in John 4:14 that the water He will give will become a *"fountain of water springing up into everlasting life."* It won't be stagnant water, but moving water with power, springing up into glory. And again, in John 7:37, Jesus says, *"If anyone thirsts, let him come to me and drink."* Again He's saying, "Just as your human body thirsts and needs water for life, I am the only one that can truly satisfy the longing in your soul." Not only can He give you spiritual refreshment as a cool drink of water, but just as water is the sustainer of all life, Jesus Christ can give you eternal life in glory.

In other stories of the Bible, God promises His people that He will always send adequate rain to bless their crops if they are obedient to Him. When He describes the Promised Land to the children of Israel in Deuteronomy 8:7, He says, *"For the LORD your God is bringing you into a good land, a land of brooks, of fountains and springs, that flow out of valleys and hills."* In their wilderness journey, God miraculously brought them water out of a rock; in the Promised Land they would never even thirst again.

Look at Exodus 40:34: *"Then the cloud covered the tabernacle of the meeting, and the glory of the Lord filled the temple."* In this particular passage and others in the Bible, the cloud symbolizes the visible presence of God, who appeared as a cloud to lead the children of Israel through the wilderness. The cloud led them on their journey and protected them by day from the scorching desert sun. When the cloud hovered over the tabernacle, they were to remain where they were and rest, whether it was five days or five years.

Whenever the cloud moved, they were to follow. The cloud assured them of God's presence.

After realizing the true significance of water for life and reading how God expresses and demonstrates this importance throughout the Bible, I decided to nickname water "glory." Of all the substances on earth, I think it's fair to say that water is one of the most glorious. No wonder God chose these spectacular droplets to represent His presence.

Glenda was a client who didn't like water at all. She drank sodas and coffee and few or no other beverages. Of course she stayed fatigued (not realizing that the lack of water causes dehydration, which causes fatigue), and she stayed constipated. She said she hated to drink water. But one day I told her this story of the glory of God showing up to the Israelites in the cloud. When I finished the story, I asked, "Have you had your glory today?" And I could see the glow on her face, then a smile.

That story changed her whole attitude toward water. When she realized that God symbolically uses water because of its importance and that God wanted her healthy, she agreed to drink it.

Today she is addicted to water, if that is possible. The change started in her mind and then she acted on it. She developed a new view of water.

Now she doesn't go anywhere without her water bottle and doesn't drink sodas and rarely drinks coffee. She eats less and no longer suffers from fatigue and constipation. Simply adding water to her diet made a significant change in her well-being.

Can you imagine each rain as being symbolic of God pouring down His glory on the earth to bring forth life? Think about this: Every time you drink a glass of water, you are pouring down the glory of God to maintain life.

There's a story in I Kings, Chapters 17 to 18, that clearly shows that the rain we automatically take for granted is truly God showing his goodness and grace and His life-sustaining power to us. Elijah was a great prophet of God. At this time, Israel had had a long line of wicked kings who didn't serve God and led the people in heathen practices and the worshiping of idols. These kings were so wicked that God would send various prophets to try to convince the people to return to God.

God sent Elijah to give a message to King Ahab, the worst king of Israel. Not only was Ahab a wicked king, but he was married to the most wicked of all women, Jezebel, who practiced idolatry and immoral behavior. She greatly influenced Ahab in wicked schemes, including killing a man for his vineyard, trying to kill all of the prophets of God who were left in the land, and leading the people to worship the god Baal. Baal was considered to be the god of the weather, including rain, so he was given credit for the people's harvests. God sent Elijah to Ahab to predict a drought in the land to let him and the people know that it is God and God alone who has the power to bring forth the rain that produces a bountiful harvest. So for several years it didn't rain, which brought drought and famine to the land. In the midst of this drought and severe famine, God sent Elijah to the Brook of Cherith, where he had water and was fed by ravens, and when the brook dried up, God sent him to Zarepath, where a widow and her son fed him and gave him a place to stay. Years later, Elijah returned to King Ahab and predicted that the rain would return and it did.

God used this demonstration to show the people that it was by His divine power alone that it rains. He is the only true and living God who has the power to stop the rain or bring it forth so there may be a bountiful harvest on earth. He is also the God who can supply all of the needs of His people in spite of a famine, as He provided for Elijah, the widow, and her son. The rain is truly symbolic of God's life-sustaining power and glory.

Have you had your "glory" today?

Water helps tremendously with weight management. In nature, water cleanses and refreshes the earth and the atmosphere. In the Bible it symbolically washes away our sins (as in baptism). Drinking water washes our bodies of harmful products or toxins. This internal cleansing is very important for overall good health and weight management.

Do not wait until you are thirsty before you drink water. Thirst is actually a warning signal that you are not drinking enough water. (If you have constant thirst, check with your doctor; it could be from taking certain medications or from an illness such as diabetes.) To avoid dehydration and to maintain proper functioning of the body, you need to create a "water cycle" to constantly replace the fluids you lose.

The first step toward developing a "water cycle" is to set a goal to drink at least eight to ten cups of water every day. The specific amount of water required varies from person to person depending on the amount of energy used daily. However, drinking eight to ten cups per day is an estimated amount to ensure you're getting an adequate supply to make up for water losses throughout the day.

When Sharon started the weight management class, she complained about feeling sluggish and thirsty all the time. She went to her physician and found out her health was fine. However, she was only drinking one or two glasses of water a day. Once she learned about the importance of water and the problems a lack of adequate water in the body could cause, she knew she had to drink more water. She started drinking more—four glasses a day—but Sharon insisted she could not drink eight glasses daily.

When I asked her what size glass she was using, she said she used a tall glass. I suspected her glass held at least sixteen ounces, or two cups. I told her to use a measuring cup to determine the size of the glass. When she returned to class the following week, she said she was surprised to discover the glass actually held two cups of water.

Sharon's mistake had been not knowing how much she was actually drinking. Be aware of the size of your container. I think most of us have our favorite glass or cup that we grab when we get a drink at home. I know I do. My favorite is actually a dainty, slender glass that holds one and a half cups of liquid, so I use it when I drink beverages such as juice, milk, or rice or soy drinks. The cup I use for herbal tea or hot chocolate holds a little under a cup and a half of liquid. My water glass holds two cups of water, so I know if I drink four of these a day, I've had my eight cups of water and my other beverages are extra.

Before I developed the habit of drinking water, I drank high-calorie beverages if I was thirsty. Usually it was a sugary juice drink, milk, Kool-Aid, or a soda every now and then. Today I know not to reach for drinks like soda, fruit cocktails and juices, Kool-Aid, and coffee to quench my thirst. Although these beverages contain water, none of them are as good for you as the real thing. When you drink plain old water, your body doesn't have to process the sugars, artificial sweeteners, or chemicals found in other drinks. Your body gets all of the wonderful benefits without all of the extra work. Water is also low in sodium, has no caffeine, and acts as a natural laxative. Those other drinks combined with my food intake contributed to my constant weight gain.

Understanding calories the way I do today, I understand why I gained so much weight. One cup of whole milk has 150 calories—and I drank at least six cups a day. That's a total of 900 calories a day just in milk!

Some alternatives to water are beneficial to you—milk or milk substitutes like rice or soy drinks (of course, low-fat)—and pure juice. With milk you get not only water but also vitamins and plenty of calcium. With juice you get plenty of vitamin C. Other foods, especially fruits and vegetables, are also sources of water. For example, two cups of lettuce is 95 percent water, and two cups of watermelon is 92 percent water.

Another thing about sodas. In addition to providing the extra calories, these drinks provide no nutrients for the body and often contain caffeine. Caffeinated beverages are not a good source for fluid because caffeine has a diuretic effect, which actually increases water loss.

Don't be deceived. Colas are not the only sodas with caffeine; 75 percent of soft drinks contain caffeine. Read the label.

Now, getting back to knowing how much water you drink: What I find very helpful in keeping track of the amount of water I drink daily—and what seems to work for a lot of other people—is to use a quart container (32 ounces/4 cups). I fill it up with water twice a day. My goal is to drink at least two of these containers, which meets my requirement of eight cups of water for the day. And believe me, when I first started drinking water it was just that to me: a requirement only. It was hard for me to drink water because I don't like cold water. Cold water is refreshing on a hot day. Other than that I prefer room-temperature water.

With so many large drinking containers and water bottles available today, don't get discouraged if you don't drink it all in a day. Starting out, you just want to try to increase your intake of water. If you have to use a straw, sip to your heart's content. Get it any way you can.

I told you earlier that this plan is about improvement. So keep striving until you make it. If you have trouble keeping track of water by the glass, try getting a large container and keep track that way. After a while you'll find that drinking water will become a habit. But remember: Your thirst is not an indicator that you need to drink water; it actually means you waited too long too drink.

In the story in John, Chapter 4, that I mentioned earlier, Jesus beautifully illustrates His plan for salvation by using thirst, an important physical function: One day Jesus was on His way to Galilee via Samaria. Although it was a shorter route to Galilee, Jews generally avoided traveling via Samaria because Samaritans weren't pure Jews; they were a mixed race resulting from the intermarriage between foreigners and Jews and were therefore hated by pure Jews.

On this day Jesus arrived at a local well around noon, where He met a Samaritan woman of ill repute. The women of Samaria came to this well to draw water twice a day, morning and evening, but this woman came at noon to avoid the other women, probably because of her reputation. Regardless of her race and her promiscuous reputation, Jesus spoke with her. He wanted to offer her the gift of salvation and caught her attention with a very crucial physical element—water. He told her the water He had to offer was "living water" and said that those who drank of this water would never thirst again. This truly caught her attention. She thought that she wouldn't have to come to the well twice every day to draw water if she accepted this water Jesus was offering, and this was good news to her.

Although she didn't immediately understand the true meaning of His message, Jesus caught her attention because she knew how significant water was in order to satisfy her thirst. She was willing to listen to what He had to say because He was talking about something she could relate to. As He continued, He told her about her life and the life God had to offer. His message really meant that He is the major source for life, the major source for satisfying that longing or craving: the thirst in her soul. She eventually realized that He must be the promised Messiah and got so excited that she dropped her water pot and ran back to the city to tell others about Christ.

Water is an abundant available resource, like the gift of salvation Jesus offers freely to all people regardless of race or past reputation. Maybe some of us would appreciate it more if we had to draw it from a well twice a day and then carry it back into the city. But just because water is now readily available to you, right at your fingertips, don't take it for granted. It must truly be an essential element for health and life, if Christ used its significance to save a soul and share the message of eternal life. So drink up!

PRAYER

Remember, you can write this prayer on an index card and keep it with you to read at those times of temptation.

Dear God,
I Corinthians 10:31 tells me that whether I eat or drink or whatever I do, do all things for your glory. I am asking you to continue to provide me with the knowledge and the determination I need to care for my health. I now know that you really care about my health, and because you care, I also care. I thank you for revealing the truth to me through illustrations in your word. And that truth is, you're concerned about my physical and spiritual wellbeing. I also thank you for water that can be so easily taken for granted. Thank you for the rain that falls to the earth, to fill it with bountiful crops that make up our food supply. I am acknowledging you right now as being the one and only God who has all power in your hands. You have the power to care for me and provide me with everything I need to live a healthy life. I'm asking you to continue to lead me and give me help in the areas where I may need it the most. Help me use the resources that you have made available. Help me remember to drink more water. Give me the desire for pure water and less desire for beverages that may not be healthy. Also, as you're quenching my physical thirst with the glorious water that you have so generously provided for me, quench my inner thirst so that I will not try to sat-

*isfy it with anything that is harmful to my health. Allow me to
truly eat and drink to your glory so that I can be all you have created me to be, a fit and healthy temple, inside and out. Amen.*

ACTIVITIES

Here are some tips that can help you create a habit of drinking
water:

1. Start your day with a glass of water. Just as it is a habit to
brush your teeth in the morning, also start your day with a glass of
water. After going all night without water, this is refreshing for the
body.

2. Drink water with meals and snacks. Get into the habit of
drinking a cup of water with your meals and snacks. If you eat at least
four to five times a day and drink water with each meal, this will account for most of the water needed for the day. Or if you use a sixteen-
ounce glass, like I do, this accounts for at least eight cups of water.

**3. Drink water when you would normally drink soda, cof-
fee, or caffeinated tea.** Caffeine has a diuretic effect, causing the
body to actually lose water through more frequent urination. The
more caffeine, the more fluid loss. You have to drink more than eight
cups of water to make up for the fluid loss.

4. Take water breaks on the job. Some people can get so involved in their work that they never stop to drink water. I had one
client who set up a program on her computer so that she received
reminders to take a water break.

5. Keep a bottle or glass of water on your desk to sip on.
Adding lemon or lime slices gives the water a nice refreshing taste.

**6. Treat yourself to sparkling water instead of other bev-
erages.** This is one of my favorite treats. I drink sparkling water over
ice, or I'll mix two parts of sparkling water with one part of 100 per-

cent juice, preferably orange juice. This is also a good alternative for people making the switch from soft drinks, because the carbonation in the sparkling water gives it a fizzing sensation.

7. Travel with a bottle of water. You can even buy a carrying case for your water bottle, and using one helped me develop the habit of drinking water because I always have water with me. Just take your bottle of water, put it in the case, put the strap on your shoulder, and you're ready to go. If you're out all day like me, fill up your bottle periodically or stop at the store and buy another bottle of water. And don't forget, when you're traveling by airplane you'll need to drink even more water. The low humidity and recirculating air within the pressurized cabin promote dehydration. (Body fluids are lost through evaporation on the skin.) This dehydration can cause fatigue and aggravate jet lag. So drink at least one cup of water for every hour you're flying.

8. Drink water before, during, and after exercise. You need to consume at least four to six ounces every fifteen to twenty minutes to prevent dehydration and muscle cramping. With dehydration the muscle loses strength and endurance, which decreases physical performance and increases risk of injury.

9. Keep your body well hydrated in the summer. Hot, humid weather causes your body to perspire more and therefore lose more water. Drinking plenty of cool water will stop the body from overheating and reduce the risk of heat-related illnesses and death.

10. Keep your body well hydrated in the winter. It is just as important to drink enough water in the winter as it is in the summer. During the winter months we spend most of our time indoors, where the heat evaporates the moisture in your skin.

If you follow these tips properly, you may have to get used to another water cycle: Frequent urination. Eventually, though, your bladder adapts to the change and you won't feel the pinch of nature so often. Anyway, urination is a good way to tell if you're drinking enough water. Clear urine is a good indicator that your water cycle is fine. Dark yellow urine means you need to drink more water (unless you're taking vitamins or medications that can darken the urine).

Don't try to do everything on this list at once and drive yourself crazy. Try one or two tips at a time, then eventually add on. Continue them until they become a habit and you feel you have to have your "glory" for the day.

One of the Scriptures that encouraged me to be "fit for God" was **I Corinthians 10:31**: *"Therefore whether you eat or drink or whatever you do, do all for the glory of God."*

God cares not only about what we eat, He also cares about what we drink, knowing that we need a constant supply of our life-sustaining beverage. Whenever you drink your water, think of it as a divine toast and say aloud or to yourself, "To God be the glory!"

Get rid of the excuses that may be stopping you from being "fit for God"

1. Lack of Discipline

Discipline is a training that is expected to produce a specific type of behavior. The more you practice living healthy, the more it will become part of your life. Make improving your health a habit with the goal of pleasing God and helping others. **I Corinthians 9:27** *But I discipline my body and bring it into subjection, lest, when I have preached to others, I myself should become disqualified.*

2. Alcohol

So many families and lives have been destroyed from the effects of alcohol. Alcohol impairs judgment and the ability to make the right decisions. It impairs speech and vision and has been the cause of many motor vehicle accidents and deaths. It can dull a person's inhibitions, making him or her more susceptible to fall victim to sin. God needs you sober and in your right mind to be an effective witness for Him. **I Peter 5:8** *Be sober, be vigilant; because your adversary, the devil, walks about like a roaring lion, seeking whom he may devour.*

3. No Plan

With the hectic schedules that so many people have today, healthier living has to be planned in order to fit it into our schedules, or most of us won't find the time to live right. Make sure you develop a plan and, as you exercise it, trust God to order your steps. **Proverbs 16:9** *A man's heart plans his way, but the Lord directs his steps.*

4. Self-Pity

Dry your tears and take a look at your cure. The remedy for self-pity is trusting in God. **Psalm 37:3–5** *Trust in the Lord, and do good; dwell in the land, and feed on His faithfulness. Delight yourself also in the Lord, and He shall give you the desires of your heart. Commit your way to the Lord, trust also in Him, and He shall bring it to pass.*

5. Physical Limitation

I am inspired when I see people commit to taking care of their health who are confined to wheelchairs, have a limb amputated, or have other physical limitations. I've had clients who could barely walk without a cane or crutches but were committed to keeping their bodies fit. If you have a condition that limits your ability to exercise, you don't have to give up on improving your health. Many health centers now have exercise equipment specifically designed for people who have physical challenges. Do what you can while leaning on God's strength to help you in your area of weakness. **II Corinthians 12:9** *And He said to me, "My grace is sufficient for you, for My strength is made perfect in weakness."*

Week Three

Eat Plenty of Fruits, Vegetables, and Whole Grains

Let the Earth Bring Forth Grass, the Herb that Yields Seed,
and the Fruit Tree According To Its Kind.

—GENESIS 1:11

According to the Book of Genesis, God created the world and everything that's in it in six days; then He rested on the seventh day. He first provided light, and then divided the waters from the waters so dry land could appear. Next He brought forth plant life from the earth. God knew that once He created man and animals they would need food, so He didn't create man, then food. He created food, then man. He made the earth, and then made it fruitful to bring forth vegetation for man and cattle.

When God described the Promised Land to the children of Israel in Deuteronomy, Chapter 8, emphasizing the abundance of water (as I discussed in Week Two), He also described it as ". . . *a land of wheat and barley, of vines and fig trees and pomegranates, a land of olive oil and honey; a land in which you will eat bread without scarcity . . .*" (Deuteronomy 8:8–9).

Just as God planned a water cycle to sustain life, He also created a food cycle. He created plants, which produce seeds, so more plants could be produced and the cycle continued. Additionally, plants produce the oxygen we breathe. Without plants, we wouldn't be able to eat or breathe. Plants also help keep the soil together so it won't be washed away by water or blown away by the wind. Isn't God awesome?

This is the same way you should think if you want to lose weight and keep it off. Be patient and plan like God did. It's important for you to get this information and learn how to apply it so you won't just obtain your new self, but you will *maintain* your new self. It saddens me when I see people so desperate to take off the weight that they diet without focusing on changing their lifestyle. I understand, because I was so desperate I didn't care how the weight came off, either. But after diet after diet and failure after failure, I had to finally accept defeat. Many others experience this same problem. As soon as they stop the diet, they gain back all the weight and maybe even more. They really don't want to take the time to learn the right way, because it's not fast enough for them. And in return for another quick fix, they again experience failure and defeat.

If you're going to lose weight and keep it off, learning the importance of foods and healthy eating will be a key factor in determining your success.

All the food we eat comes from plants. As a matter of fact, grass is the first plant God mentions. The grains we eat are from the seeds of grasses. Bread and pasta are made from the kernels of wheat, which starts out as a green grass that dries out in the sun and changes color to a golden brown. So whenever you eat a sandwich, a slice of pizza, or a plate of spaghetti, just remember that grass from the earth made it all possible.

How many fruits, vegetables, or whole grains have you had today? It never fails: Whenever I teach a weight management class or work with clients individually, most people agree that they eat few or no fruits, vegetables, or whole grains, yet these foods are vital for our overall well-being. Our bodies need the elements contained in these foods for proper functioning and for optimal health. The problems we have with obesity and many of the diseases we see today could be prevented, or the risk greatly decreased, just by including these natural foods in the diet.

The American Heart Association and the National Cancer Society agree that a diet plentiful in these foods decreases the risks of obesity, heart disease, and certain types of cancer and other illnesses. So what do these foods contain that are so important?

In the Book of Daniel, we meet Daniel, a Hebrew prophet deported by King Nebuchadnezzar of Babylon when the king captured Jerusalem. Daniel and three of his friends were taken to Babylon to serve in the king's palace. There they went through an intensive training program to be taught the culture, language, and literature of the Babylonians. The Babylonians had tried to change the thinking of Daniel and his friends by giving them a Babylonian education. They tried to change their loyalty to their Hebrew culture by changing their names. All of the young men selected to serve in the king's palace had to eat the food and drink that the king appointed for them. This was because the king wanted all of those serving him to look healthy as well as be intelligent and well versed in their culture.

But Daniel, though in a new culture, still held firm to his religious beliefs and didn't want to defile himself with the king's delicacies and drink. So Daniel asked one of the king's servants if he and his three friends might not eat of the royal food and delicacies appointed by the king. The servant said he feared the king and didn't want to be blamed if Daniel and his friends looked worse than the other young men in the palace. But Daniel knew there was something valuable about natural foods. He knew if God made it, he did not have to worry about his health.

He asked the king's servant to put him and his three friends to the test. Let them eat only vegetables and drink water for ten days, then examine their appearance. If he was not satisfied with their appearance, he could do to them whatever he saw fit. If Daniel and his friends were not healthier than the others in ten days, they would be in danger of losing their heads.

At the end of the ten days, Daniel and his companions looked healthier than all the other young men. So the king's delicacies were taken from the other young men and all of them had to eat vegetables.

I can remember my sister LaReese having to sit at the table long after we all finished dinner because she wouldn't eat all of her vegetables. She had a hearty appetite. But she just wouldn't eat her vegetables. She and Dad had their own daily battle, and the rest of us patiently and silently waited to see who the winner would be for the evening. Meanwhile, she had to remain at the table, and my Dad sat next to her until she finished all of her vegetables. She was so determined not to eat them that many times my father just threw up his hands in frustration and gave up for that evening, until they went through the next round of the fight on the following day.

I thought to myself: She wouldn't have to go through all of this if she just did what I did. Before I got my plate, I grabbed plenty of napkins and put them in my lap. As I ate my vegetables, I frequently wiped my mouth, folding the napkin and putting it in my lap. When I was done—or when everyone thought I was finished eating—I quietly got up from the table and headed immediately for the bathroom.

I am so surprised that my parents never knew the truth. Of course, I was dumping my food from the napkins.

You may be able to relate to my story of me at the dinner table. You've heard for years that natural foods are good for your health and important for weight management, but for whatever reason you still do not include them in your diet. I'm convinced that losing weight and improving health are truly personal choices. You won't succeed if you do it only to please others or just for a quick fix. Look at what the Bible says about Daniel in Daniel 1:8, *"But Daniel purposed in his heart that he would not defile himself with the portion of the king's delicacies . . ."* Daniel didn't just provide lip service like so many people do month after month, New Year after New Year, decade after decade. Something happened inside of him. He was surrounded by people drinking all kinds of beverages and eating all types of foods, just as many of us are at work, at church, or at family events, but in spite of his surroundings he purposed in his heart that he was going to live healthy. The Amplified version of the Bible says, *"He determined in his heart,"* and the Living Bible says, *"He made up his mind."* It starts with the way you think, a thought of determination in your mind that will eventually manifest itself on the outside.

David so strongly believed in eating right that he was willing to give not only his life but also the lives of his friends. He knew from experience, because he ate healthy and therefore was in good health. This is what happened to me. I finally decided that if these foods were good for me and helped me lose weight, then I would find ways to include them in my regular diet. I was tired of feeling sluggish and not having any energy. I was tired of my emotional roller-coaster ride of feeling good or bad depending on my "food fix" for the day. And when I did select healthy food choices, I felt so much better. I made up my mind that I was going to stop neglecting my body and was going to lose weight and be healthy. But I had to first get the knowledge and understand why these foods were important for my health.

Likewise, it's important for you to know why these foods are so important. Knowing how the essential nutrients found in natural foods work in your body and why they are important will help you understand *why* you need to eat healthier.

Six nutrients are needed to maintain proper functioning of the body. They are: water, carbohydrates, vitamins, minerals, protein, and fats. And although fiber is not a nutrient, it is also essential for proper functioning of the body.

1. WATER

Water is the most basic nutrient needed by the body and has many functions in it, as discussed in Week Two. Many natural foods such as fruits and vegetables contain water. Remember that, for example, two cups of lettuce is 95 percent water by weight, and two cups of watermelon is 92 percent water by weight. Even a medium baked potato with skin is 71 percent water by weight.

2. CARBOHYDRATES

Carbohydrates supply the fuel or energy to move, think, and operate effectively and efficiently. Did you ever go a period without eating and then feel lightheaded, get a headache, or not be able to think anymore? This occurs because your body is running out of fuel. Energy foods such as grains, cereals, nuts, vegetables, fruits, and legumes are all parts of plants.

Although there are two classifications of carbohydrates—sugars and starches—the body cannot tell them apart. Simple sugars, such as the fructose found in fruits, are digested more quickly in the body because they can be absorbed as they are. Complex carbohydrates, such as in a baked potato, have to be broken down in the body into a simple sugar before they can be absorbed from the digestive tract into the bloodstream to be used as energy.

Both sugars and starches supply the body with four calories per gram of carbohydrate. Unfortunately, the starches—such as bread, cereal, pasta, and rice—are the carbohydrate foods that have been falsely labeled as a dieter's nightmare. Some vegetables, like the baked potato and sweet potato, contain a high percentage of complex carbohydrates and have also been mislabeled. Many people try to avoid these carbohydrate-rich foods when they want to lose pounds; often, the real problem is too many carbohydrates or portions that are too large. Another problem is what most people put in or on the food that makes it so fattening; it's all the butter, sour cream, gravies, and sauces that add extra calories to these foods. Avoiding carbohydrates in your diet is like not putting gas in your car when your gauge is on empty and you need to get to work.

When I was desperate to lose weight, I stayed away from them, too, only to find myself unable to function at my best and too weak to exercise. Then I found out that these foods were my main energy supply, and that my weakness and light-headedness were caused by trying to exclude them from my diet. Contrary to what most people think, many of these foods are low in fat, and they are loaded with the vitamins, minerals, and fiber necessary to keep the body functioning properly and minimize the risks of illness and disease.

3. VITAMINS

Vitamins regulate chemical reactions within the body. They include vitamins A, B complex, C, D, E, and K. Vitamins don't provide energy for the body, but they are essential for life. Without them our bodies do not function properly. For instance, without vitamin A you cannot see in dim light; without vitamin C you are susceptible to diseases and illnesses because it enhances the immune system, and so on.

Not only do vitamins help certain metabolic reactions take place within the body, but they also serve as antioxidants, which help prevent diseases. Vitamin C, vitamin E, and the carotenoid beta-carotene (a precursor to vitamin A) are antioxidants; they protect cells against free radicals that can cause cell damage, thus increasing the risk for disease.

Although oxidation is a natural process that takes place with age, according to recent studies, most of the illnesses we experience as we get older may occur from the free radical damage to cells. Antioxidants neutralize the free radicals, serving as a defense or protection for the cells. I'm sure you've heard that to prevent a cold you should take plenty of vitamin C, and for healthier skin and to reduce wrinkles or fine lines in the skin you should use creams and lotions containing vitamin E. It is possible that these antioxidants also have a vital role in the prevention of illnesses such as heart disease, certain cancers, and other diseases of aging.

The body does not manufacture most vitamins. They are best

when absorbed from natural foods that are eaten rather than when taken as a supplement. Fruits, vegetables, and whole grains are loaded with vitamins. Many fruits such as oranges, grapefruits, strawberries, tangerines, kiwi, and cantaloupe are good sources of the antioxidant vitamin C. Vegetables are excellent sources of vitamin C and beta-carotene in addition to many other nutrients. Vegetables generally have a higher nutritional content than fruits and also contain phytochemicals, which are substances found in plants that protect against diseases.

Cruciferous vegetables, or those in the cabbage family, such as cabbage, cauliflower, kale, broccoli, collards, and others, are believed to provide protection against cancer. The deeper yellow and green vegetables, such as broccoli, spinach, carrots, and sweet potatoes, have more beta-carotene.

Whole grains such as whole wheat bread and brown rice or other whole grain products such as wheat germ and cereals are excellent sources of the B vitamins. Whole grains, as well as nuts—another plant food—also contain the antioxidant vitamin E.

Now you can understand why Daniel and his three friends, eating only vegetables, were healthier than all the others in the king's palace. By living off of vegetables it was as though they were taking vitamin pills daily. Because these vitamins came from natural foods, the nutrients were better absorbed and used by the body.

When God was leading the people of Israel to the Promised Land, in Numbers, Chapter 13, Moses sent spies ahead to bring back a report about the land. He sent men who were heads of all the tribes and told them to go and see what the land was like. He also told them to bring back fruit from the land. He wanted to know if the land was rich and fertile with a plentiful harvest of the nutrient-rich foods. And just like God said, it was a land full of natural, wholesome foods. The men brought back grapes so large they carried them on a pole between two of them. They also brought back pomegranates and figs. This was definitely a land in which the people could thrive and live in abundant good health because of these nutrient-rich foods from the earth.

4. MINERALS

When you hear the word "mineral," perhaps you think about rocks in the earth. But minerals for the body are essential for life. Like vitamins, minerals help regulate many bodily functions such as fluid balance, muscle contractions, and nerve impulses. They also contribute to the body structure.

There are two classifications of minerals: major minerals and trace minerals. The major minerals are not more important than the trace minerals; they are just needed in greater amounts in the body. Major minerals include calcium, magnesium, phosphorous, and potassium. Trace minerals include chromium, copper, iodine, iron, and manganese.

Again we see God's wisdom in planning. Not only do minerals help regulate bodily processes, but they also help form structures in the body. According to Genesis, Chapter 1, God created man from the earth and He brought forth plants from the earth. Plants use minerals from the earth to help them create the food they need to grow; in turn, we must eat the plant foods that contain minerals in order for our bodies to grow and function properly. For instance, calcium gives structure and strength to bones and teeth. Bones and teeth contain 99 percent of the calcium found in the body. Although dairy products such as milk, cheese, and yogurt (which we will talk about later) are rich sources of calcium, calcium is also found in green vegetables such as broccoli, bok choy, and kale. Many juices, such as orange juice, are now fortified with calcium, and the citric acid from the juice helps increase the absorption of calcium. Osteoporosis, a disease that causes weakness of the bone, making bones more susceptible to fractures, is caused by a deficiency of calcium.

Iron, another important mineral, is found mostly in the hemoglobin of red blood cells. Iron is an essential part of hemoglobin that carries oxygen-rich blood to every cell in your body. I'm sure that you have heard of anemia or iron deficiency, especially in women due to our regular menstrual cycles. Symptoms of iron deficiency can include an increase of infections and increase the risk of infections and fatigue or weakness. Iron is found in foods of animal origin (as will be discussed later) and foods of plant origin. Some good plant sources of iron include soybeans, peas, whole grain breads and cereals, leafy green vegetables such as spinach, red kidney beans, lima beans, and prune juice.

Many of the natural foods are good sources of the minerals needed for good health. To ensure you're getting an adequate amount of the necessary nutrients, it's important to eat a variety of foods. Not all the substances in foods have been discovered yet, so when you eat the food source you're getting the good stuff we know about and good stuff we don't know about yet.

5. PROTEIN

Protein is known as the building material of the body because it makes up the structure of every living cell. Protein helps regulate body processes, repairs body cells as they are damaged or wear out, builds and repairs muscle, and, as antibodies, protects you from bacteria and viruses that can cause illnesses and disease. Protein also supplies the body with energy if you don't eat enough carbohydrates. However, eating adequate carbohydrates saves the protein so it can perform its important function to repair and build body tissue.

Protein is very important for health and weight management, especially if you want to develop a sleeker, more toned, shapelier body. Protein is responsible for developing the muscle tissue needed for the tighter, firmer figure. When I used to think of protein sources, meat always came to mind. (Meat can be considered natural because God made it, but we're specifically referring to plant foods.) Animal sources are complete proteins because they contain all of the essential amino acids, the building block for proteins. However, the concern with consuming too many animal foods is fat, because generally meat has a higher fat content than foods of plant origin. (I'll discuss eating meat in more detail later, in Week Five.) People who eat a diet consisting mostly of foods of plant origin tend to eat less saturated fat and cholesterol (found in animal products), eat more fiber, and consume more phytochemicals.

Remember, in the Book of Genesis, God is preparing the earth to be inhabited by man. He created food first, then man, and then in Genesis 1:29, He says, *"See, I have given you every herb that yields seed which is on the face of all the earth, and every tree whose fruit yields seed; to you it shall be for food."*

According to this statement, I can assume man was originally a vegetarian because God didn't mention him eating meat until after the flood in the days of Noah. Almost all foods of plant origin contain protein, except for fruit. No one plant food contains all the essential amino acids; therefore, plant foods are incomplete proteins. The soybean is the only plant food that is complete. In other words it contains all of the essential amino acids, or "building blocks." Some people call it God's gift to the earth. That's why today you hear more and more about foods from the soybean, such as tofu, soy milk, and many other products.

Vegetarians get sufficient protein by eating a variety of vegetables, grains, legumes, nuts, seeds, and fruit. The body needs the combination of amino acids for a complete protein. If an amino acid is lacking in one food, you can get it from another. Variety is the key. Am I saying become a vegetarian? No. That is a personal choice and, praise God, He gave us choices. However, if you don't eat meat, poultry, or fish, then dairy products (milk, yogurt, and cheese) and eggs are also good sources of protein. If you don't eat any of these foods, variety is key to ensure that you are getting sufficient protein.

Good plant sources of protein include nuts, peanut butter, tofu, hummus, and beans. In addition to eating a variety of foods, you can combine some foods to create a complete protein: a peanut butter sandwich, pasta and cheese, beans and rice, milk and cereal, a cheese sandwich, and a tortilla and beans are some good combinations.

6. FAT

It's a shame that because of our concern with being overweight, fat most often has a negative connotation. Fat is not a bad word. Fat is an essential nutrient, one you can't live without.

It is not realistic to say you want "a fat-free diet." Fat has many vital roles in the body. For instance, the fat-soluble vitamins, A, D, E, and K, cannot be used to nourish the body without fat carrying them in the bloodstream. Fat also combines with other nutrients to form important compounds in the body. Certain fatty acids help children grow properly and are also needed for adults to have healthy skin. Fat helps regulate body temperature by providing insulation for the body. A layer of fat around our internal organs helps cushion and protect them from injury; and fat also supplies energy for physical activity.

Fat itself is not the problem when it comes to being overweight. Consuming *too many* high-fat or high-calorie foods is the problem. Fat calories are a concentrated calorie source and if you don't burn them off, or if you eat too many, fat is stored in the body under the skin.

One of the major benefits of eating a diet rich in fruits, vegetables, and whole grains is that these foods are naturally low in fat. Animal fats, which are generally high in saturated fat, can contribute to heart disease, certain cancers, and other illnesses.

7. FIBER

You should also eat more fruits, vegetables, and whole grains because they are excellent sources of fiber. Although fiber is necessary for good health, fiber is not a nutrient because it is cannot be converted into energy like carbohydrates, proteins, and fats, and it is not used for bodily processes as vitamins and minerals are. Then why is it important? High-fiber diets decrease constipation, reduce the risk of colon cancer, and even lower blood cholesterol levels.

As you see, natural foods provide many wonderful benefits to promote health for the body, but we have to increase our intake of natural foods in order to reap the full benefits God intended.

One of my absolute favorite stories in the Bible is the story of Ruth in the Book of Ruth. The Book of Ruth is an eloquently written story of how a Moabite woman joined God's people out of her love for her mother-in-law, Naomi. Her virtuous character, strength, and hope won her a place among God's people and favor with God. Ruth is one of the most encouraging books of the Old Testament. It shows that in spite of hardships and struggles, if you trust God, He will never fail.

Naomi left her home of Bethlehem with her husband and her sons to move to Moab. While she was there her sons married; however, Naomi's husband and both of her sons eventually died. Naomi decided to return to her home of Bethlehem, which means the "city of bread." She encouraged her daughters-in-law to go back to their homes with their families, but Ruth refused to leave her and became committed to follow her and serve Naomi's God, the God of Israel. Ruth and Naomi returned to Bethlehem, the "city of bread," empty-handed. They didn't have anything, not even food to eat.

Naomi was now old, so Ruth chose to go out in the fields with the reapers to glean. Gleaning was when the poor were allowed to pick up leftover grain that had fallen to the ground during reaping. Day after day Ruth went out in the fields, in the midst of the heat, bending over, picking and picking to collect enough grain for her and Naomi to have a meal for that day. The only thing most of us have to do today is jump in the car and drive to the store and purchase wholesome foods. We don't have to use much energy; it only requires a desire to eat better. If we had to go out into the fields in the heat of the day and pick up pieces of grain as they fell to the ground, we would have a deeper appreciation of what God has made so readily available to us.

Ruth's story doesn't end here. Because of her hard work, determination, and willingness to do what was right in the eyes of God, her devotion was well rewarded, physically and spiritually. God led her to the field of Boaz, a godly Hebrew man who accepted a kinsman's responsibility and married Ruth, ending her days of hardship. God also used this Moabite woman to give birth to Obed, who was the grandfather of the greatest king in Israel's history, King David. Therefore Ruth became an ancestress of our Lord and Savior, Jesus Christ. Despite the fact that Hebrews weren't allowed to associate with people of Moab, because the people of Moab were idol worshipers who sacrificed their children and burned them on the altar, Ruth's faithfulness and willingness to trust God were well rewarded.

God clearly shows in this story that He does not discriminate among people. His love and help reach out to all people who are willing to trust in Him. Will you trust Him and begin to do what's right for your body?

Maureen was a client who rarely ate any natural foods. She was significantly overweight, suffered with constipation, and was always tired and lethargic. Her typical menu was: for breakfast, some type of high-fat muffin or donut and a cup of coffee; lunch was a greasy burger, fries, and soft drink from a fast-food restaurant; and then she had a dinner of processed food made out of a box, followed by her midnight snack of cookies or chips.

I found this to be pretty typical of many people struggling with losing weight. Her diet was lacking significantly in the proper nutrients needed for optimum health. She had more than enough calories, but they were mostly empty calories, having no real nutritional value. She didn't drink enough water or eat high-fiber foods; therefore, she suffered with constant constipation. The thought of eating vegetables was like eating grass, she said.

Maureen did fine with Week One and Two. She journaled and recorded her positive thoughts and daily food intake, and she began drinking plenty of water. The change called for in Week Three was difficult. She was skeptical. It took patience on my part. I explained repeatedly why these foods are so important and slowly her outlook changed. I also started with something personal to Maureen.

She often took laxatives and was thinking about getting a bowel cleansing for her frequent constipation. Instead of her doctor taking the time to discuss her diet with her or recommending a nutritionist, the doctor just recommended various types of laxatives and the cleansing. I explained to her that one of the important functions of natural foods was to aid in waste elimination. Fruits, vegetables, and whole grains contain fiber, which aids in the removal of intestinal waste.

Today, Maureen eats a whole grain cereal or oatmeal with fruit for breakfast most mornings, and she also includes fruits and vegetables in her diet daily. She now eliminates waste regularly without a laxative, snacks less, and lost weight by adding this week's step into her lifestyle. She is no longer hungry all the time, her mental outlook and self-esteem have improved, and she is more energetic.

It took creative experimenting and planning, but eventually eating healthy became part of her daily life. Instead of snacking on chips, cookies, and donuts, she eats more of nature's sweets: fruits. Her family and friends were totally shocked to see the tremendous improvement in her eating habits, weight, and energy level at only Week Three.

So how do you ensure an adequate intake of these substances? We need a plan. We're still imitating God. He had a plan and we need a plan as well.

The Department of Agriculture and the Department of Health and Human Services developed the Food Guide Pyramid, which you have probably seen on food containers.

The Food Guide Pyramid is an outline of foods you need to eat daily to help you plan, and it determines whether you're getting sufficient nutrients and calories. It is a good visual aid to help you assess your dietary intake and help you make healthier food selections. The pyramid consists of five food groups: the bread, cereal, rice, and pasta group; the vegetable group; the fruit group; the milk, yogurt, and cheese group; and the meat, poultry, fish, dry beans, and nuts group. Oils and sweets are listed as a category rather than a group. The government agencies list recommended servings for each group. The foods are grouped together because their nutrient contents are similar.

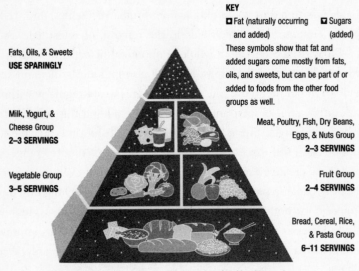

KEY

☐ Fat (naturally occurring   ☑ Sugars
     and added)   (added)

These symbols show that fat and added sugars come mostly from fats, oils, and sweets, but can be part of or added to foods from the other food groups as well.

Fats, Oils, & Sweets
USE SPARINGLY

Milk, Yogurt, &
Cheese Group
2–3 SERVINGS

Meat, Poultry, Fish, Dry Beans,
Eggs, & Nuts Group
2–3 SERVINGS

Vegetable Group
3–5 SERVINGS

Fruit Group
2–4 SERVINGS

Bread, Cereal, Rice,
& Pasta Group
6–11 SERVINGS

SOURCE: U.S. Department of Agriculture/U.S. Department of Health and Human Services

The government chose to use a pyramid-shaped structure to house the food groups rather than the square used for the "basic four food groups" because it better represents the proportion of foods needed in your diet from the bottom up. The foods at the bottom or largest portion of the pyramid (bread, cereal, rice, and pasta) are needed in the greatest amount, versus the foods listed at the tip of the pyramid, which are needed in the least amount or sparingly (fats, oils, and sweets). Because this program is all about God, let me make another spiritual connection here.

Egyptian pyramids were built to protect the body of a person so that the person's soul would be preserved forever, according to Egyptian religious beliefs. Indians used pyramids as places for their temples.

According to the Bible (I Corinthians 6:19–20), your body is a temple of God. When I think about the Food Guide Pyramid housing the different food groups needed for sufficient nutrients, I think about the temple, representing the body, which needs these specific foods for good health.

The triangular sides of the pyramid are symbolic also. A triangle is the symbol used to represent the trinity of God (God the Father, God the Son, and God the Holy Spirit). A pyramid has triangles all around it; therefore, eating right is all about being at your best so you can be all God created you to be. This is my personal interpretation to keep me focused on taking care of my body, God's temple.

In biblical days the temple was also the place of worship. We now call our place of worship "church." Would you mistreat in any way the church, which is the house of God? Would you throw trash and garbage up and down the aisles? Your body is the house of God and it is precious in His sight. He wants you to be a fit temple all around, inside and out. Start by using the pyramid as a guide to eating a variety of healthy foods.

Let's review the first three food groups listed in the pyramid, because the natural foods I'm discussing in this step are included in these food groups located at the base of the pyramid. The other food groups will be discussed in Week Five.

BREAD, CEREAL, RICE, AND PASTA GROUP

I mentioned earlier that we get the most important food in the world from grass or the seeds of grasses. And the foods listed at the very bottom of the pyramid—bread, cereal, rice, and pasta—are all foods made from grain, the seed of grasses. These foods are excellent sources of complex carbohydrates, the body's chief energy source. They help gas up our engines. Because grains are plant foods, they are naturally low in fat (remember, it's what you put on them that makes them high in fat) and rich in nutrients. If eaten in the form of a whole grain (without the nutrients removed through processing), these foods supply the body with the mineral iron, which is important for healthy blood, and B vitamins, which help your body use the energy from foods.

Whole grains are also good sources of fiber. Although these foods are listed at the bottom of the pyramid, you don't want to load up on too many refined products such as white bread, pasta, and rice, which have lost much of the natural fiber and nutrients during processing. You need to include whole grains and cereals in this food group so that you can get sufficient nutrients and fiber to promote good health and prevent constipation.

Just as today, in biblical times grains were used in almost everything eaten. They were naturally good choices when compared to other foods, because unlike vegetables, milk, and meat, grains can be stored for a long period of time without spoilage. During their journey in the wilderness, God fed the people of Israel an unusual food called "manna," which was also known as "bread from heaven." In Deuteronomy, Chapter 8, when God described the Promised Land to the children of Israel, He told of a land full of grains, where they could eat bread without scarcity.

Jesus Christ says in John 6:35 and 6:48, *"I am the bread of life,"* and in John 6:51, *"I am the living bread."* In other words, He is the main energy source for those who believe and trust in Him. He is the sustainer of life, the spiritual bread that will satisfy our every desire on earth and give us eternal life in heaven. When we eat physical bread, however, we have to continuously eat it to supply our daily energy requirements. Jesus is saying that He is spiritual bread that will satisfy our every desire on earth and give us eternal life in heaven.

In the Book of Genesis, during the seven years of famine in Egypt, Joseph stored plenty of grain so that the nation would not die of starvation. People from other lands traveled from afar to Egypt to purchase grain. Grain was so important that it was also used as money in trading. This shows not only the importance of grain but also the importance of careful planning. Joseph saved an entire nation of people by careful planning. Learning the plan will help you make better food selections.

The recommended number of servings from the bread group per day: 6–11. If you eat ½ cup of oatmeal for breakfast, a sandwich (with 2 slices of bread) for lunch, several small crackers as a midday snack, and ½ cup of rice and a small roll for dinner, you've eaten six servings.

Most people eat more than this because their servings are usually larger. For instance, a bagel, a large roll, or a muffin can be two to three servings each. Examples of a Bread Group Serving (per the American Dietetic Association):

- 1 slice enriched or whole grain bread (1 ounce)
- ½ hamburger roll, bagel, pita bread, or English muffin
- 1 (6-inch) tortilla or 1 cup cooked rice or pasta
- ½ cup cooked oatmeal, grits, or Cream of Wheat
- 1 ounce ready-to-eat cereal
- 3–4 small crackers
- 1 (4-inch diameter) pancake or waffle

Many people try to avoid the bread group when trying to lose weight, especially with all of the low- or no-carb diets. But if you really check out the truth, you'll discover that in most cases it's not the carbs that are the problem; it is how much of them you eat, what you put on them, and what time you eat them. Eating large portions and loading them with butter, gravies, and sauces will add on the pounds. Extra calories in the body turn into extra pounds on the body. And eating a meal with a large serving of carbs in the late evening or at night isn't helpful either. This is the time of day when the body winds down, and you don't need all of the extra energy. So again, if you have any extra energy at the end of your day, it will be stored as extra fat on your body.

In biblical days bread was a very important part of the meal. It was so important to life that Jesus used it to explain the most important and most profound spiritual concept in the Bible—His death and resurrection. This was the whole purpose for Jesus coming to earth, to die for the sins of the world. So as He sat in the upper room in Jerusalem the night before His crucifixion with His disciples, He used bread to symbolically represent His body that would be broken and bruised for our sakes. He instituted the Lord's Supper by breaking the bread, blessing it, and telling His disciples to eat it, as it represented His body.

The Lord's Supper is such an important part of Christian fellowship today that churches all over the world, regardless of denomination, regularly partake of it. The Lord's Supper, or Communion, is a provision of bread and fruit of the vine that Christians partake in remembrance of what Jesus did on the cross. Christ used bread to symbolize His body because, just as He is the main source for eternal life, bread was the main energy source for people during that time. Once again God used something that people understood to teach this great spiritual truth. If bread was good enough for Jesus, it's good enough for me. However, I try to eat only whole grains and, just like with anything else, it's important not to overdo it.

VEGETABLE GROUP

The next food from the bottom up in the pyramid is the vegetable group. Some of the vegetables mentioned in the Bible are leeks, onions, cucumbers, garlic, mustard, and mallows. Before the children of Israel entered the land of Canaan, the Promised Land, they were given instructions in farming so they could produce a variety of healthy crops.

Most of us don't produce our own crops, but eating a variety of vegetables for health is important. The nutrients vary in each vegetable. Deep yellow vegetables such as carrots and sweet potatoes and dark leafy green vegetables such as spinach and kale are good sources of the antioxidant beta-carotene, which can protect you against cancer. Tomatoes and bell peppers are good sources of vitamin C, and dry beans and peas are good sources of fiber. (Although dry beans and nuts are plant foods, they are listed in the meat group in the Food Guide Pyramid.)

Again, it's not these natural foods that are fattening, but how they are prepared that can make them high in fat. French fries, a salad drowned in oily salad dressing, a baked potato covered in butter and sour cream, and greens cooked with pork are examples of good foods with too much added fat.

The recommended number of servings per day: 3–5. Examples of a Vegetable Group Serving (according to the American Dietetic Association):

- $\frac{1}{2}$ cup chopped raw, nonleafy vegetables
- 1 cup of leafy, raw vegetables (lettuce, spinach, watercress, or cabbage)
- $\frac{1}{2}$ cup cooked vegetables
- $\frac{1}{2}$ cup cooked legumes (beans, peas, or lentils)
- 1 small baked potato (3 ounces)
- $\frac{3}{4}$ cup vegetable juice

FRUIT GROUP

As discussed earlier, fruits are good sources of vitamins A and C. Berries, melons, and citrus fruits such as oranges, tangerines, and grapefruits are rich in vitamin C, and deep yellow fruits such as cantaloupe, mangoes, peaches, and apricots are good sources of vitamin A. Fruits can also supply the body with fiber, potassium, and folic acid. Fruits are low in calories, have little to no fat, and are cholesterol-free. Fruits are nature's fast foods because they can be eaten easily with little or no preparation. They also can satisfy your "sweet tooth" because they contain a natural sugar, fructose.

I believe God made fruit to satisfy man's "sweet tooth." When

God made man and placed him in the Garden of Eden, the Bible says that the garden was filled with trees pleasant to the sight and good for food. God told Adam in Genesis 2:16–17 to eat freely of every tree in the garden except the tree of knowledge of good and evil. In other words, Adam had plenty of fruit available to satisfy his sweet tooth. If you have a sweet tooth that contributes to some of those extra pounds, try eating nature's snack foods.

God also described the Promised Land as being plentiful in fruit. In biblical times grapes, figs, pomegranates, apples, dates, raisins, and olives were popular. Figs were a very popular fruit of that day, eaten fresh or dried or even used in making cakes.

One day while Jesus was walking with His disciples, He grew hungry and wanted some of nature's fast food. He attempted to get a fig from a fig tree. When He saw that the fig tree was not producing any fruit, He cursed the tree and it never produced fruit again (Mark 11:12–14).

How many fruits have you had today? Whether you have or haven't eaten any fruit today, I have another question I want you to consider: Have you produced any fruit?

"Fruit" has a very significant meaning in the Bible. A fruit is defined as having seed within itself to produce more fruits (not just fruit, but an entire tree), and the characteristics that Christians should have are called "fruits." These fruits are produced by God's Holy Spirit and are described in Galatians 5:22–23. They are love, joy, peace, longsuffering, kindness, goodness, faithfulness, gentleness, and self-control. The Bible refers to them as "fruit" because you ought to be able to produce more and more, enough for yourself and for you to share with others.

Which fruit would you like to produce in your life? Maybe you need more kindness toward others, or maybe you need more self-control to avoid overeating. Whatever fruit you need, you can ask God to give it to you and He will. As I told you in the very beginning,

God is right there to assist you, guide you, and direct you. So I'll ask you again: Have you had some fruit today? Have you shared some fruit with others? Make sure you get both the physical fruit that's good for your body and the spiritual fruit that's good for your soul.

The recommended number of servings per day: 2–4. Examples of a Fruit Group Serving (per the American Dietetic Association):

- 1 medium fruit (apple, orange, banana, or peach)
- ½ grapefruit, mango, or papaya
- ¾ cup juice
- ½ cup berries or cut-up fruit
- ½ cup canned, frozen, or cooked fruit
- ¼ cup dried fruit

There are really no "bad" foods. All foods can be incorporated into a healthy lifestyle if eaten in moderation. But I believe you also need to know what you're eating. There is some truth to the statement "You are what you eat." If all you eat is fattening, salty, high-calorie foods, then you have fat, salt, and a high level of calories entering your body, and it can show, inside and out, through illness, fatigue, or being overweight. If you eat foods that are low in fat and loaded with nutrients and phytochemicals, then you have these health-promoting substances in your body, and it probably shows inside and out by having a healthy-looking body. You really need to understand that when you don't eat these foods, it's like putting clothes in the washing machine without any detergent. The machine is rotating or moving, but the clothes are not being completely cleaned.

Eat plenty of fruits and vegetables (at least five servings per day)

Let's review a serving of fruit and vegetables:

$^{1}/_{2}$ cup fruit

1 medium-size whole fruit

$^{3}/_{4}$ cup fruit juice

$^{1}/_{2}$ cup cooked vegetable

1 cup leafy greens or salad

$^{1}/_{4}$ cup dried fruit

$^{1}/_{2}$ cup cooked beans

Please don't make *drastic* changes in your diet. This program is about making gradual changes until they become part of your lifestyle. It takes time, commitment, and consistency for success. Remember, the characteristics that Christians are to possess are called "fruits." A fruit starts out as a seed, then it grows. Not only does it grow, but it can also produce more fruit. So start out gradually, and then grow naturally so that you can develop permanent lifestyle changes. Set small goals, accomplish those, and then move on. This way you'll see some progress and be able to say, "That's good," like God did after each of His accomplishments toward His new creation.

Here is a nutritional breakdown to help you plan your daily menu:

1. Eat at least one vitamin-A-rich food every day

Foods rich in vitamin A are the deep yellow fruits and vegetables and the deep green vegetables. Apricots, cantaloupe, mangoes, peaches, sweet potatoes, carrots, broccoli, collards, spinach, kale, and turnip greens are some common examples.

2. Eat at least one vitamin-C-rich food every day

Citrus fruits (such as oranges, tangerines, and grapefruits) and melons and berries are rich in vitamin C. Examples of vegetable sources of vitamin C include the dark leafy green vegetables such as broccoli, collard greens, kale, and spinach to name a few.

3. Eat a vegetable from the cabbage family (cruciferous) at least several times per week

Cruciferous vegetables or vegetables from the cabbage family have been connected with cancer prevention. The name "cruciferous" is derived from their four-petal flowers, which look like a crucifer, or cross. They include bok choy, broccoli, brussels sprouts, cabbage, cauliflower, collards, kale, kohlrabi, mustard greens, radishes, rutabaga, turnip, turnip greens, and watercress.

Here are some practical tips to help you include at least five servings of fruits and vegetables in your daily menu:

1. Buy a variety of fruits and vegetables. Buy fresh, frozen, dried, and canned fruits and vegetables. When buying canned fruit, make sure it is not packed in heavy syrup, which adds on the calories. Buy canned fruits in their natural juices.

2. You've heard the saying "Out of sight, out of mind." Keep fruits and vegetables in sight so that you can easily grab them when you need a quick snack. Keep fruit that doesn't need refrigeration in a bowl on your kitchen table or counter, and keep cut-up vegetables in a container on the top shelf of your refrigerator. Keep them in sight so you won't forget them.

3. Drink a glass of 100 percent juice, such as orange juice, with your breakfast or as a midday snack.

4. Eat fruit with your breakfast. Put banana or raisins in your cereal or top your pancakes and waffles with fruit such as strawberries, blueberries, or apples.

5. Mix low-fat yogurt with fresh fruit as a snack, or put fresh fruit such as strawberries in a flan or dessert shell and top with whipped cream for dessert.

6. Put fruits or vegetables on a sandwich. Try lettuce, tomato, cucumbers, sprouts, peppers, apple, or pineapple. When packing for lunch, place fruits and vegetables in a separate plastic bag so your sandwich won't get soggy.

7. Include vegetables in your lunch such as celery, broccoli or cauliflower florets, cherry tomatoes, or carrot sticks.

8. Eat more salads. Load your fresh garden salad with more vegetables, or make an all-fruit salad using your favorite fruits. Create a "combination salad" including a variety of both fruits and vegetables. In addition to the fruit salad, one of my favorite salads is the pasta salad. I'll include fresh vegetables such as carrots, tomatoes, cucumbers, broccoli, or some of my other favorites with pasta and a low-fat Italian salad dressing. When eating salads, don't defeat the purpose of eating low-fat by loading your salad with dressing in which 90 percent of the calories comes from fat. Use low-fat or reduced-calorie salad dressing. When eating out, ask for your dressing on the side so that you can control the amount in your salad. Don't include high-fat foods in your salad, which also defeats the purpose of eating low-fat. Eating more salads is a great way to eat a variety of fruits and vegetables, and eating a large salad is a great way to get many of your suggested servings for the day.

9. When making a roast, soup, or stew, load up on the vegetables.

10. Make a pizza with pizzazz. Add steamed vegetables and cut back on the cheese. Try broccoli, mushrooms, tomatoes, zucchini, spinach, onions, red and green peppers, or shredded carrots. You can try almost any of your favorites on pizza and in many other dishes.

11. Add vegetables to your omelet. Include onions, peppers, tomatoes, broccoli, or any other of your favorites.

12. Add chopped vegetables to dishes such as lasagna, meat loaf, and spaghetti.

13. Try baking with fruit. Add applesauce, bananas, or peaches in recipes for baked goods such as pancakes, homemade bread, and muffins. One of my favorites is adding bananas and raisins to bran muffins or, for variety, I'll also make bran muffins with apples, raisins, and cinnamon. Mashed or pureed fruit adds great flavor and gives a smoother texture to the food.

14. When you eat at restaurants, fill up on fruits and vegetables instead of bread. Order a side dish of vegetables and try fruit for dessert.

15. Take fruit for lunch. Include an apple, orange, peach, tan-

gerine, grapes, cherries, dried fruit, a banana, a box of raisins, or other fruits in your lunch bag. Keep them handy in your office or in your briefcase for a quick snack, too.

16. Drink fruit juices instead of sugary drinks and sodas. Try even mixing different juices to create a different great-tasting drink.

17. Make stir-fry with a combination of vegetables.

18. Eat larger portions of vegetables and fruits.

19. At fast-food restaurants, order a fresh salad and a baked potato.

20. For convenience, choose fruits and vegetables that require little to no preparation or chopping such as apples, grapes, baby carrots, broccoli spears, bananas, raisins, and cherry tomatoes.

I won't say "Don't eat sweets." But foods high in sugar and fat contribute to unwanted pounds. Fruits taste great, have nutrients for the body, are low in calories and fat, and are cholesterol-free. Try some of these ideas if you are a big sweet eater like I was.

Here are some of my favorite healthy desserts:

1. My absolute favorite is my fruit shake or fruit smoothie. I put fruits such as strawberries and bananas in a blender with ice and low-fat milk or low-fat yogurt. I also enjoy smoothies with fruit juice, which gives the drink an entirely different taste. Adding milk to a smoothie creates more of a milk shake; juice gives it a more fruity taste. Again, experiment. Add vanilla, cinnamon, nutmeg, and other flavors until you find what satisfies you.

2. Fruit slush. I put a blend of my favorite fruit juices—maybe pineapple and orange—in the freezer, and take it out before it freezes completely.

3. Frozen fruit pops. Pour juice into ice pop or ice cube trays and you'll have a healthy fruit pop for you and the kids. It costs less to make fruit pops than to buy them from the supermarket, and there's no sugar added.

4. Frozen fruit pieces are also a nice treat. Take banana slices or seedless grapes, place them in a plastic bag in the freezer and you'll have a nice frozen fruit treat.

5. Instead of drinking sodas, try adding fruit juice to sparkling water over ice. This is a really refreshing drink that helped me make the transition to healthier drinks. The carbonation of the sparkling water adds a nice fizz to the natural fruit flavor.

Striving to eat five fruits and vegetables a day doesn't have to be challenging. I'll share some of my actual entries from my journal to show you how it can be done. I hope you are keeping a food journal by now and are committed to writing in it, because you're going to need it throughout the book.

MY JOURNAL ENTRY FOR FRUITS AND VEGETABLES

Breakfast:	a glass of orange juice
	a banana
Snack:	
Lunch:	an apple
Snack:	
Dinner:	carrots
	broccoli
Snack/Dessert:	strawberry fruit shake

On this particular day I met my requirements for "five a day," vitamin A, vitamin C, and a cruciferous vegetable. On another day I added another vegetable by eating a salad for lunch.

Eat whole grain breads and cereals (at least three servings per day)

Here are some tips for including more whole grains in your diet:

1. Choose breads, rolls, muffins, and bagels made from whole grains such as whole wheat, cracked wheat, multigrains, or oats rather than those made from white flour, which is poor in fiber. Read the label. Just because a bread is brown doesn't mean it is whole wheat or from a whole grain. Whole grain breads are browner than bread made from white flour; however, some bread is brown because of the caramel coloring added, which is listed on the food label. The ingredient listed first on the label is present in the greatest amount. Make sure the first ingredient is mainly whole wheat or another whole grain flour.

2. If you can't imagine switching from white bread to wheat, try toasting the wheat bread before you eat it until you get used to the taste. This helped me make the change. I ate wheat bread in the morning with a little margarine and fruit spread, and it tasted pretty good.

3. Try making whole wheat pancakes and waffles. You can start by using both white flour and wheat flour to make them. If that's the best you can do, that's still healthier than using white flour only.

4. Select a whole grain cold or hot cereal such as bran flakes or oatmeal for breakfast. Add nutritious fruit.

5. Try adding whole wheat flour to some of your baking recipes. Try at least half whole wheat flour. Again, it requires some experimenting to find out what works for you.

6. Try a whole wheat pita. Pita bread has a pocket, so you can use your imagination and stuff it with some of your favorite foods—tuna fish, chicken, or vegetables. My favorite is using the pita and adding some of my homemade pizza fixings.

7. At least once or twice a week use brown rice and whole wheat pasta instead of white. Alternate for variety, or use them together.

8. Eat crackers made from whole grains. Read the label to make sure they are not high in fat.

9. Add wheat germ to hot cereal, cold cereal, pancake and waffle

mix, yogurt, soup, salads, lean ground beef or turkey, stuffings, baking mixes, and many other foods.

10. Create your own snack mix using whole grain cereals, broken pieces of pretzels, peanuts, and raisins.

John 6:5–13 tells how a great multitude of people followed Jesus because they were amazed at His miracles and His ability to cure diseases. Jesus realized that before taking care of their spiritual needs, He had to meet their most basic need—food. He asked one of his disciples, Philip, *"Where shall we buy bread that these may eat?"* Philip immediately assessed the cost because they needed a great amount of money if they were going to feed over five thousand people. They were helped when they found two small fish and five barley loaves (barley is a natural grain).

After Jesus blessed the food, He gave it to his disciples to distribute. Miraculously, every single person was fed, and there were even leftovers. Matthew 15:32–38 recounts how Jesus miraculously fed over four thousand people with bread and fish, and again there were leftovers. Jesus wanted to teach His disciples that He was able to supply the most basic human needs in addition to meeting their spiritual needs.

How many grain foods did you eat yesterday or today? Look at your food journal. Here is an example of one of my journal entries with the bread group only, including whole grains:

Breakfast: a bowl (1 cup) of oatmeal
Snack:
Lunch: 2 slices of whole wheat bread
Snack:
Dinner: ½ cup rice
Snack: several wheat crackers

Eating healthy requires some planning, but it isn't as difficult as some think. It requires more effort in the beginning, but with consistency your plan and schedule become part of your daily routine. Before you know it, eating healthy is a habit just like brushing your teeth in the morning. You'll find yourself reaching for that piece of fruit.

I have not only developed the habit of drinking two glasses of water every morning before my day starts, but I also eat a banana and drink a glass of orange juice. It is such a part of my life that I absolutely have to have bananas. I find myself taking bananas with me when I stay overnight at workshops or conferences. I've even taken boxed orange juice with me as well. My point is, I started out making a conscious effort to eat natural foods; then after a period of time, it just became a habit and I began to do it automatically.

Maureen, the client I mentioned earlier, began by adding a salad to her lunch every day. Eventually she included more natural foods in her daily diet. She did it the right way, making gradual changes that were realistic for her. Set small goals, accomplish those, determine your room for improvement, then add on more goals, more natural foods. If a farmer plants watermelon seeds, he expects watermelons. If he plants an apple seed, he expects an apple tree. If you mistreat your body by not eating properly, then why be surprised when you get ill?

Do you expect a harvest of good health, or is there room for improvement?

PRAYER

Remember, write this prayer on an index card so you can read it whenever you need to:

Dear God,
I thank you for giving me the knowledge to care for my health.
I really want to live a healthy life. I know that I have talked

about it over and over, but this time help me with the change that needs to take place on the inside of me. Help me to purpose in my heart a refusal to continue to neglect my body. I have made up my mind that I will lose weight; I will feel great and I will be energetic, vibrant, and alive. I will take advantage of all of the wonderful natural foods you have made available to me— fruits, vegetables, and whole grains. Forgive me for taking them for granted. Give me the desire to eat more natural foods, and give me the patience for gradual changes that will become a permanent part of my life. Keep me focused, as you kept Daniel focused on pleasing you by taking care of his body. Amen.

Study Scriptures

GALATIANS 5:22–23

But the fruit of the Spirit is love, joy, peace, longsuffering, kindness, goodness, faithfulness, gentleness, self-control. Against such there is no law.

JOHN 6:51

I am the living bread which came down from heaven. If anyone eats of this bread, he will live forever; and the bread that I shall give is My flesh, which I shall give for the life of the world.

ACTIVITIES

Use your journal

- Record how many fruits and vegetables you eat today (at least five). Did your food choices include a fruit or vegetable rich in vitamin C (such as citrus fruits or juice); high in vitamin A or dark yellow (such as cantaloupe, sweet potato, or carrots); or a dark green, leafy vegetable or a cruciferous vegetable from the cabbage family?

- Record how many whole grain breads or cereals you have eaten (two to three servings).

- Write a plan for improvement with some of the tips for consuming more fruits, vegetables, and whole grains I shared in this step. Make gradual, realistic changes that you can keep. You can always add more later.

- Shop at a market that sells fresh fruit or vegetables, or visit a farm to pick your own. Plant a small garden of your own. Or if the weather or season doesn't permit any of this, go to a health food store or the health food section of your supermarket to discover new items. Try new fruits and vegetables you haven't eaten before. Variety is the key for good health.

- If weather permits, participate in a new outdoor activity this week. Some outdoor activities include gardening, biking, hiking, or swimming. If you don't know what to do, get outside and wash your car. Scrub, wash, wipe, and shine until your heart is content. Remember to switch arms so that both arms get a great workout. If you have more than one car, make it a family event and get others involved.

- Replace one of your normal high-calorie snacks with one of the recommended fruit snacks this week.

- Many church groups go on collective fasts for various reasons (fasting doesn't have to mean abstaining from *all* foods). But in many instances the true intent of a fast is not accomplished. People fast, then afterward overindulge and neglect their bodies, creating unhealthy lifestyle practices. Is God truly pleased with the fast when His desire is for us to also be in good health? If you belong to a group that fasts, encourage them to go on an "unnatural food" fast. This means giving up foods that are not natural such as candies, pastries, high-fat foods, sugary drinks, and products made with white flour. Eat only natural foods (whole grain products, fruits, vegetables, and 100 percent fruit juices; meat is optional). This will serve a dual purpose: accomplishing the purpose of the fast by abstaining from foods that God didn't create from the earth, and teaching people how to care for their temples and develop healthy eating habits. This will also cleanse the body of all of the harmful toxins or by-products found in processed foods. Note: Meat and dairy products are optional, but high-fat dairy products such as ice cream, whole milk, and cheese should be avoided. Also, high-fat meats such as beef and pork should not be eaten during the fast. If meat is eaten, it should be limited to fish and poultry, and should not be fried.

During this type of fast you'll be able to focus spiritually on your intended purpose of fasting in addition to learning how to appreciate and enjoy the natural foods God has made available to keep the body functioning properly and in good health.

Get rid of the issues that may be stopping you from being "fit for God"

1. "FAST FOODS ARE MORE CONVENIENT"

America has more fast-food restaurants than most other countries. We also have a higher rate of obesity and heart disease. Fast foods can be quicker and more convenient than cooking, yet in addition to convenience you are paying for extra calories. And calories in the diet show up as extra fat on the body. Although all foods, including fast foods, are okay in moderation, eating them daily is not good for your health. Whatever you put in your body will eventually show, whether it does so through illness or significant weight gain. **Galatians 6:7–9** *Do not be deceived, God is not mocked; for whatever a man sows, that he will also reap. For he who sows to his flesh* *will of the flesh reap corruption, but he who sows to his Spirit will of the Spirit reap everlasting life. And let us not grow weary while doing good, for in due season we shall reap if we do not lose heart.*

2. "I'm just too busy"

There is a story in Luke 10:38–42 about Jesus and two sisters named Mary and Martha. Jesus came to visit Martha's home. Mary, her sister, sat at Jesus' feet and listened to his words, but Martha was distracted, busy in the kitchen preparing to serve. Martha got agitated because Mary wouldn't help her, so she complained to Jesus. Jesus' response to her was, *"Martha, Martha, you are so worried and troubled about so many things. But one thing is needed, and Mary has chosen that good part, which will not be taken away from her."* With the everyday cares, concerns and goals we have in life, we can get lost and distracted with doing so much, so that like Martha we miss what's really important. Martha really thought that it was important to serve Jesus food, but Mary decided to sit at His feet and listen to His words. She wanted to know more about Him; she wanted a personal relationship with Him. She wanted to know His voice, His ways, and what pleased Him. Many people, especially those of us in the ministry or otherwise working in the house of God, get so busy working to "serve" God that we are just too busy to get to know God. Other people who are not involved in church functions are so busy that they also miss what's really important in life. You may be too busy to get to know that good part, that part that no one can take away from you—the peace of God, the joy of God, the power of His Holy Spirit to give you self-control in the time of need; His awesome love that fills your heart and mind so that your light can shine and you can share His love with others. Spending quiet time with God in His word and in prayer is the only way to get to really know Him. When you choose to sit at His feet, as Mary did, and get intimate with Him, you'll discover He cares about every aspect of your life. **I Thessalonians 5:23–24** *Now may the God of* *peace Himself sanctify you completely; and may your whole spirit, soul, and body be preserved blameless at the coming of our Lord Jesus Christ. He who calls you is faithful, who also will do it.*

3. LACK OF KNOWLEDGE

If you cannot spare the extra funds to join a health club or invest in a personal trainer, there is still no excuse. You can find good exercise books and videos everywhere, and there is plenty of fitness information on the Internet, in magazines, and on television programs. Don't allow bad eating habits to destroy you. Get the knowledge. **Hosea 4:6** *My people are destroyed from lack of knowledge. Because you have rejected knowledge, I also will reject you from being priest for Me; because you have forgotten the law of God, I also will forget your children.*

4. CIGARETTE SMOKING

Nicotine is a very addictive and dangerous drug. It also increases the risk for illnesses such as heart disease, lung cancer, and various respiratory conditions. Secondhand smoke is also unsafe. Use wisdom and allow God to strengthen you to kick the habit or to lead you to the right help. **I Corinthians 3:16–17** *Do you know that you are the temple of God and that the Spirit of God is in you? If anyone defiles the temple of God, God will destroy him. For the temple of God is holy, which temple you are.*

5. FEELINGS OF INADEQUACY (OR, YOU FEEL LIKE YOU CAN'T DO IT)

In reality, you are inadequate if you rely on your own strength and ability. The Bible clearly tells us that our sufficiency for all things comes from the one who is all-sufficient. Trust in God to help you and allow His Spirit to strengthen you in the time of need. **II Corinthians 3:5–6** *Not that we are sufficient of ourselves to think of any thing as being from ourselves, but our sufficiency is from God, who also made us sufficient as ministers of the new covenant, not of the letter but of the Spirit; for the letter kills, but the Spirit gives life.*

Week Four

Now Is the Time to Exercise!!!

Let There Be Lights in the Firmament of the Heavens to
Divide Day from Night; and Let Them Be for Signs and
Seasons, and For Days and Years.

—GENESIS 1:14

During the fourth step of creation (Genesis 1:14–19), God created order in the universe. He made the sun, moon, and stars. He created the sun to rule the earth by day and the moon to rule or govern the earth by night. This gave us our time— days, years, and seasons. God didn't need time because He is eternal. But He was planning for humankind to be maintained on earth, and we need this order and time for our survival.

For instance, man is able to live on the earth because the sun is the right distance from the earth. If the earth were too close to the sun, we would burn up and die; if we were too far from the sun, we could freeze to death.

Can you imagine what your life would be like if God hadn't given order to the earth? One moment it could be dark, then light; it could be snowing, then one hundred degrees, and so on. We wouldn't even know our own age or the ages of our children. We wouldn't know when to prepare for rain, snow, or hail, not to mention floods, tornadoes, and hurricanes. It would be chaos. That is how it feels when many of us get on the vicious cycle of yo-yo dieting.

Consider my experience: One moment I was on one diet program, then I was on another. I tried this pill, then that shake, then the next diet, and so on. My weight constantly fluctuated. I kept a variety of different clothes sizes in my wardrobe because I didn't know what size I would be from one day to the next. My emotions were on a roller coaster. I didn't know if the next diet would cause irritability, stomach cramps, or dry mouth; have me bouncing off the walls because of the caffeine, or have me walking around like a zombie due to lack of energy. I was completely out of order. My life was chaos.

But God is awesome. Just as He created order in the universe, He is giving you the opportunity to stop this vicious cycle and create order as well. No matter what diet programs you tried in the past, no matter how many times you failed, no matter how hard it's been for you to lose weight and keep it off, do you really believe you can fail with the help of a God who is incredibly strategic and awesome in His creation and planning?

God didn't look at His world in its chaotic state and give up, and you don't have to, either. He took a chaotic world and created order. We need to imitate Him by creating order in our lives as well.

Thank God for revealing the truth about who He is and showing us His omnipotence and sovereignty, for He is the Almighty God and Creator who cannot fail. I thank Him for letting me know I can do all things with Him.

The earth is constantly moving. It spins like a top on its axis as it travels simultaneously around the sun. These two movement patterns determine our days and years. It takes about 24 hours for the earth to spin around its axis once. This spinning movement is what gives us our night and day. It takes about $365\frac{1}{2}$ days for the earth to travel completely around the sun, which gives us our year.

Just as the earth moves in three ways—on its axis, around the sun, and with the rest of the solar system—the human body was also made to move in more than one way. Without movement you and I cannot live. Every single molecule in the body moves. Our lungs expand and deflate involuntarily. Our heart muscles contract to pump blood from the heart to the rest of the body. Even when we eat, the muscles in the esophagus move to push down food. Waste elimination takes place through muscular contractions of the intestinal walls. Electrical impulses travel throughout our bodies to control heart rate, breathing, the release of hormones, and other movements of the body. There is a lot of moving going on inside us to maintain order for life, but we also need movement on the outside to maintain order for weight management and optimum health.

Year after year I hear people blame their weight on getting older or on having children. Now that I am a little older and have three children, I feel I can say it's time for us to stop giving these reasons for our weight gain. Although it's true that for every ten years of age your metabolism decreases, this is a slight decrease and should not have a significant effect on your weight. And yes, I absolutely ballooned in weight when I had children, but really, being pregnant wasn't the true culprit; it was what I put in my mouth. The pregnancies seemed like a valid excuse for me to eat for two. The problem was the lack of order or balance. I ate more calories than I burned off.

Remember, initially God brought order to a chaotic earth by putting some things in place. For each extra 3,500 calories we consume, we gain an additional pound. We also need order if we want to keep what we have in place. Those extra calories are stored in the body as fat. If we continuously consume more energy or food than we expend or burn, we will continuously gain weight.

According to the *American Journal of Sports Medicine,* two-thirds of all Americans are dieting, and most will fail because they are not combining caloric reduction with exercise. Exercise is a missing component. Experts and researchers agree that exercise is a necessary component for good health. That is what gives order or balance to our health.

The American Heart Association (AHA) has identified physical inactivity as a major risk factor for coronary heart disease. The Centers for Disease Control and Prevention (CDC) recommends that all Americans accumulate at least thirty minutes of moderate-intensity physical activity on most days, preferably every day of the week.

I lost weight on each diet I tried, but could not keep it off once I returned to normal eating. You can lose weight on almost any diet. *Maintaining* the weight loss is the problem. Statistically, nine out of every ten dieters gain the weight back in the first year. I believe part of the reason is that the focus is on weight loss and not on a healthy lifestyle or a maintenance program.

Although many Americans consume too many calories, the lack of activity or a sedentary lifestyle is a major culprit as well. As we get older we become more sedentary. When many of us were children or teens, we ran outdoors, rode our bikes, went skating, participated in some organized neighborhood activities or sports teams, went to parties, and so on. Even if you just walked to the park or through your neighborhood or to the playground with your friends, you moved more.

Then somewhere in our mid to late twenties or early to mid thirties (it varies from person to person), we gradually became more settled in our careers and families, and did not move around as much.

My client Cecilia was at a conference for women when two girlfriends decided to take the stairs from the lobby to the third floor instead of waiting for the elevator. To Cecilia's surprise, she was leaning on the handrails and gasping for air before they reached the third floor. She huffed and puffed. Her heart beat hard and fast. Sweat ran down her face.

This experience changed her life. Although she ate a pretty healthy diet and always wanted to lose ten to fifteen pounds, she didn't think it was absolutely necessary to exercise because she looked nice in her clothes. She attributed the extra ten to fifteen pounds to getting slightly older and therefore accepted it as natural.

Cecilia didn't realize that the purpose of exercise is not just to look a certain way or have a slimmer, firmer body, but that it is also about being able to perform the daily activities of life with greater ease. After the expereince with the stairs, Cecilia began to exercise regularly. With time and consistency, her stamina improved and she lost ten pounds.

Eating well without exercising is like having a beautiful new car in great operating condition and no gas. The parts all work, but you can't go anywhere. Just as cars are built for transportation or movement, or just as the earth rotates or travels around the sun, the human body was also made to move. Movement of the car helps keep the engine and other parts in good working order, movement helps keep the universe in order, and the human body also needs movement to maintain its order.

Most people years ago ate whatever they wanted to eat. Many of the jobs we have today contribute to the problem. People sit at computers for eight to ten hours a day, and the only exercise they get is walking back and forth from the house to the car and from the parking lot to the office. The only toning exercise many people do is the "push-away," pushing away from the table after eating. We don't even get up to change television channels anymore.

Life is too full of conveniences. We have no reason to get up and move. We can even shop for household goods or buy our groceries on the computer.

But exercise is a key component for weight reduction and weight management. God is a God of movement. He is a God of action. In the very beginning, before God spoke creation into existence, in Genesis 1:2, the Spirit of God was moving over the earth.

The people of God in the Bible moved. There was nothing sedentary about the people of God in biblical days. Unlike many workers today, people in biblical times had very physically demanding jobs and they exerted a lot of energy. For example, it was common for the people of Israel to keep herds of sheep and goats. Many shepherds wandered from place to place to make sure their herds had sufficient water and food. This was a very hard job that required staying outside for the most part, tending the herd, and protecting it from danger.

God told Abraham, the father of the children of Israel, to pack up his wife and all of his stuff and just go. Abraham did not know where he was going. He did not have a car, truck, bus, or plane, but began traveling to an unknown land with everything he owned. The people of Israel had to be in good physical condition to wander in the wilderness for forty years. I believe their grueling work as slaves in Egypt gave them the stamina they needed to survive in the wilderness while wandering around. Then when it was time for them to possess the Promised Land, God told Joshua, "... *arise, go* ..." In other words, "Get up and go."

The workers of biblical times *had* to be active. When the Israelites settled in Canaan after being in bondage to and then leaving the Egyptians, farming became a very popular way of making a living. Farming is not easy work, either, and it was harder in those days because they didn't have the equipment and irrigation systems available to modern farmers. In Jesus' time, carpenters built and prepared lumber for architects and shipbuilders, made tools, and built furniture and structural elements of houses, like doors.

God's people of old moved their bodies. The prophet Elijah outran a chariot, Samson killed three thousand men with a donkey's jawbone, and King David was a great man of valor and a warrior who killed lions and bears as well as a nine-foot-nine-inch-tall giant. He also led thousands of men in war. Deborah was the only female judge of Israel and a great leader who marched with the Israelite army, leading them in war against enemy troops.

Thank God for His grace and mercy. Thank God for His Son, Jesus Christ. Thank God for deliverance. Many of us say we want to be just like Jesus, but remember, Jesus had a walking ministry (as I call it). He and His disciples walked from town to town, up and down hillsides, and from city to city. In the Book of Acts, Philip, one of Jesus' followers, also outran a chariot. Other disciples, apostles, and followers of Jesus traveled near and far to spread the Good News.

When Jesus gave the great commission, He told His disciples, in Matthew 28:19, *"Go therefore, and make disciples of all the nations, baptizing them in the name of the Father and of the Son and of the Holy Spirit."* Many Christians today would not be able to walk down the block and would not think of going from nation to nation.

Look at II Corinthians 6:16: *"And what agreement has the temple of God with idols? For you are the temple of the living God. As God has said: I will dwell in them and walk among them. I will be their God and they will be my people."*

What would God find if He came to live in your body right now? Are you grieving His Holy Spirit? Is God suffocating or locked up, unable to be completely free in your life because His house is out of order?

Our goal in Fit for God is: To have a positive attitude, drink plenty of water, eat whole grains, and exercise.

Throughout this book I give certain Bible verses to study, but I do not claim to be a great Bible scholar. I delight in studying God's word and learning Scriptures because they have encouraged me through many of my battles. I encourage you to study the entire messages—not only the verses quoted here—to truly get the full meaning of the passages.

In I Timothy 4:8 there is a Scripture that is often misquoted or misinterpreted by people. It reads, *"For bodily exercise profits a little, but godliness is profitable for all things, having the promise of the life that now is and of that which is to come."* I've heard some Christians use this verse as an excuse not to exercise. Because it states that exercise profits a little, they say it is not important, but they miss the rest of the message.

When Paul wrote this letter to Timothy, whom he often refers to as his son, Paul was addressing some of the issues raised by false teachers in the church where Timothy was a church leader. Rather than living godly lives, these false teachers made stringent rules for the body to make themselves appear righteous (I Timothy 4:1–4). Paul addresses these concerns and says in verse 4 that all food is good as long as it is received with thanksgiving and prayer. He continues to tell Timothy how to recognize these false teachers by their doctrine, and he emphasizes the importance of godly living when compared to everything else, including exercise. He's saying there is some benefit to exercising the body, but that the greatest exercise we can get is spiritual exercise, which leads to eternal life.

Another place where physical health is mentioned in the Bible is in III John, verse 2, where John writes to Gaius, an elder in the church. John was concerned for Gaius's physical and spiritual well-being. At the time, people often overindulged in the body's sinful nature, feeling that it was okay because the body was not important.

III John, verse 2, reads, *"Beloved, I pray that you may prosper in all things and be in health, just as your soul prospers."* This Scripture or passage really speaks for itself. It clearly shows that God is concerned about our body and soul. Therefore, we should work on having both our bodies and souls "fit for God."

Because the Bible says the body is the temple of the Holy Spirit of God (I Corinthians 6:19–20), it only makes sense for us to have a fit body. When God created man from the dust of the earth, He breathed His Spirit into man's nostrils and man became a living being. The body houses the spirit and soul of man in addition to the Spirit of God. Your body is a vehicle and transports the part of us that is connected to our Maker.

All throughout the Bible, spiritual things are described by using physical examples. In Psalm 19, verse 5, the great joy of the sun is described by saying that *"it rejoices as a strong man to run its race."* This illustration is used because people took pride in athletic competitions and could relate to this example. A runner approached the competition rejoicing and excited, with the image of winning in his mind. Look at exercise the same way. Be excited in advance, with the image of the results you want in your mind, knowing that your commitment will turn it into reality.

The U.S. Department of Health and Human Services has developed a national campaign called Healthy People 2010. The goal is to improve the quality of life for all Americans through health promotion and disease prevention. The campaign includes ten objectives, or Leading Health Indicators, to help people reach this goal. The first two major public health concerns in the United States, the agency says, are lack of physical activity and obesity.

Do you need more reasons to exercise? Here are twenty ways in which you benefit from exercising regularly:

1. Exercise improves the condition of your heart and lungs. The heart is the most important muscle in the body because it pumps oxygen-rich blood and nutrients to every cell in the body. Exercise makes both the heart and lungs more efficient and stronger. The heart has to work less when it operates efficiently, thus placing less stress on this life-sustaining organ. For instance, one of the reasons many people are not able to walk up stairs without breathing hard is that the body is trying to consume more oxygen, so the heart has to pump harder. People who exercise regularly can walk up stairs and perform other daily activities without becoming short of breath because their hearts have to work less. Because their hearts have to work less, people who exercise regularly generally have lower blood pressure and pulse rates than those who do not.

This is what physical fitness is really about—being able to perform daily activities with greater ease.

2. Exercise reduces the risk of various illnesses and diseases. Research shows that regular physical activity can decrease the risk of diabetes, hypertension, heart disease (America's number one killer), and certain types of cancers. It can lower blood cholesterol levels and decrease the risk of other illnesses associated with sedentary lifestyles.

3. Exercise increases muscular strength. Physical activity such as weight lifting or muscle toning increases muscle fiber, making muscles stronger, thus increasing the body's ability to do work with greater ease. You are able to carry groceries, lift a small child, or move other items with less effort.

4. Exercise improves muscular endurance. You have more stamina and do not tire as easily.

5. Exercise will help you lose weight. Exercise helps you burn extra calories and unwanted pounds through the exertion of energy. When you burn more energy than you have consumed, you lose weight.

6. Exercise increases your metabolism. Increase in metabolism means that you burn calories or energy at a higher rate or quicker than someone who does not exercise. Someone with a higher metabolism can eat more than someone the same size, without gaining weight. Your body will burn fat even when you are not exercising or while you sleep.

7. Exercise shapes, tones, and firms your body. By burning unwanted fat and improving muscular tone, exercise improves physical appearance and creates a slimmer, shapelier, healthier-looking body.

8. Exercise helps you increase and maintain lean body mass. One of the problems with weight loss programs is that you lose lean body mass or muscle tissue while you are trying to lose unwanted fat. Exercising on a weight loss or weight management program helps you keep or build lean body mass, which is responsible for a healthy, fit, toned body. Muscle burns more calories than fat because it requires more energy to be maintained.

9. Exercise improves your posture. When the muscles are stronger and firmer, the body is erect rather than slouched over or out of alignment. Improved posture and stronger muscles can also decrease the risk of lower back pain, a common ailment as people age.

10. Exercise increases bone strength. Weight-bearing activities such as running, walking, and weight lifting strengthen the bones, which decreases the risk of osteoporosis, a condition that causes fractures and brittleness in the bones.

11. Exercise helps reduce depression, stress, and anxiety. Many doctors prescribe regular physical activity for depression because it is a natural antidepressant and tranquilizer. Endorphins or hormones released during exercise have a very calming effect. God gave us a natural tranquilizer!

12. Exercise helps reduce the symptoms associated with PMS and menopause. Again, because of the hormones released during exercise, physical activity is the alternative to drug therapy for some women who suffer with various mood swings, pain, irritability, and other physical symptoms associated with these conditions.

13. Exercise can improve your mood. Because exercise relieves tension and makes you feel more confident, it can also give you a more positive attitude.

14. Exercise helps you keep off the weight. Studies show that most people who diet gain the weight back within the first year. Those who remain physically active are the most successful at keeping off the weight.

15. Exercise can help you to eat less. Some people think if they start exercising they will have a tremendous appetite, but to the contrary, exercise can actually suppress the appetite in some people. This was true for me because I ate due to stress and anxiety. Exercise helped to relieve some of these feelings; therefore, I snacked a lot less. Exercise also seems to create a healthy mind-set; therefore, you want to eat less and select healthier food choices.

16. Exercise can help reduce medical expenses. People who exercise regularly and take care of their health tend to be ill less often than those who don't exercise.

17. Exercise can reduce job absenteeism and improve job performance. Again, people who take care of their health and exercise are absent from their jobs less frequently due to fewer illnesses. Job performance may also improve because of the benefits exercising has on the body and mind.

18. Exercise helps you sleep better. It relaxes the body and mind, which can help you go to sleep easier and sleep well.

19. Exercise helps you improve athletic performance. Physical activity improves your cardiovascular capacity, muscular strength, and endurance in various sports activities.

20. Exercise improves the overall quality of your life. I'm not going to tell you that if you exercise you'll live longer, but I know you'll feel better. Research shows that exercise allows you to feel younger longer. Regardless of how long you live, taking care of your health allows you to live a more productive, healthier, more energetic life instead of a life of suffering and pain. According to research, most of the illnesses we see today can be prevented by healthy lifestyle changes.

When I think about the benefits of exercise, cigarette smoking comes to mind. I have met many people who exercise yet continue to smoke, as if exercising cancels out the damage of smoking. Of course, it doesn't work that way.

According to Proverbs 12:1, if you get knowledge and choose not to use it, that is not an intelligent decision, and God wants us to act in wisdom. Although my father accepted Jesus Christ as His Lord and Savior and his entire life changed, he still suffered unnecessarily and died prematurely because he did not do all he could to care for his health. My father was active and had a lean, muscular build, but he also smoked most of his life and it finally caught up with him.

I never want to see another human being suffer like that again in my life. This very youthful-looking, fun-loving, strong man was reduced to weighing seventy pounds and wearing diapers, unable to do anything for himself. According to the American Cancer Society, an estimated 85 percent of lung cancer cases are caused by cigarette smoke. Smoking also increases the risk of cardiovascular disease (heart attack, stroke, high blood pressure, and other heart disorders) and cancer of the throat, mouth, lips, pancreas, stomach, kidney, bladder, larynx, and cervix. It increases the risk of chronic lung disease (emphysema and bronchitis) and also increases the risk of cancer for anyone around you who inhales the tobacco smoke secondhand.

So you should avoid being around the smoke from other people's cigarettes. And do not apologize for removing yourself from the presence of someone who is smoking. If someone was holding a gun in front of you, threatening to wound you or take your life, would you apologize for not wanting to get shot?

Proverbs 6:27–28 reads, *"Can a man take fire to his bosom, and his clothes not get burned? Can one walk on hot coals and his feet not be seared?"* **When you smoke you are literally playing with fire. Watch out; you just might get burned.**

I once saw an American Cancer Society poster that read something like this: "If smoking showed on the outside of you, would you smoke?" It had a picture of a woman whose face and hair were saturated with dark, sticky, greasy tar. I was horrified. That poster needs to be everywhere—in stores, malls, restaurants, and schools.

———

My sister has a wonderful testimony of how she was delivered from cigarette smoking by trusting in God. As matter of fact, it includes some of the same principles I use in this book. She first made the decision to stop. She wanted to care for her health because her body was the temple of God, and God's desire for her was to live a healthy and productive life. Because she was addicted and didn't know how she would stop, she quoted and believed what the Bible says in Philippians 4:13: *"I can do all things through Christ who strengthens me."* She sincerely prayed for God to take away the desire to smoke. She prayed to cleanse her body from all of the harmful effects of smoking.

One day she smelled cigarette smoke and it was sickening to her. Her desire to smoke was gone—and it never returned. She didn't try any of the products they have on the market to help her stop smoking. She didn't need a support group or a program. She made up her mind and relied on God. As the Bible repeatedly shows: He never fails.

Maybe you need a program or product. It doesn't matter. What is important is to pray and ask God to give you the desire, the strength, and the method you need for success.

Here are some practical tips on how to live a more active lifestyle. As with every other step, work at your own pace and make realistic, gradual changes.

Perform both aerobic and weight resistance exercises for maximum health benefits

Aerobic exercise is considered any activity that uses the major muscle groups in the body. It is rhythmic in nature and can be performed or maintained continuously for a prolonged period of time. Examples of aerobic exercise include walking, jogging, running, stationary and road cycling, aerobics and step aerobics, rowing, biking, cross-country skiing, hiking, inline skating, and roller-skating. The cardiovascular and respiratory systems (including heart and lungs) play a major role in aerobic activity. One of the major benefits of aerobic activities is the improvement of the ability of the cardio-vascular system to deliver oxygen to the body. Before you start any physical fitness program, remember to consult your physician.

Health experts recommend performing aerobic activity at least three to five days per week. One to two days a week will not produce significant improvement in aerobic fitness, although this amount does maintain some type of fitness level. Still, if you do not exercise at all and one to two days a week is all you can start out with, that's great. It's better to do something and strive for improvement than to do absolutely nothing at all.

One of the biggest mistakes beginners make is exercising too hard. Exercise does not have to wear you out to be effective. In fact, moderate intensity gets the best results in weight loss. Be aware of your exercise intensity.

One of the methods we use in aerobics classes to determine intensity is to find the target heart rate. The simple way to determine intensity, though, is to take the talk test. Just try talking while exercising. If you're out of breath and gasping for air, slow down. If you can talk normally and exercising is a breeze, pick up your pace.

This is a simple and effective way of determining whether you are overexerting yourself during exercise. It is also very important to listen to your body. How do you feel? Can you pick up the pace? Do you need to slow it down, or can you remain at the same pace? Increase your intensity gradually.

Aerobic exercise should be performed for at least fifteen minutes to improve aerobic endurance. For more significant improvements, exercise from thirty to sixty minutes. If you don't have a lot of time to exercise (which is most of us), or if you just want to remain healthy and in fairly good shape, try twenty to thirty minutes at least three to four times a week. This allows you to experience reasonable health gains. I normally tell my beginners (those who don't exercise at all or haven't in years) or those who are significantly overweight to do less than fifteen minutes if that is all they can do.

You'll also see benefits from short bouts of activity like walking around your block, walking your dog, or walking around your building during lunchtime. This short activity can still be motivating and mentally uplifting as you strive to get healthier.

So remember:

1. Strive to work out three to five days per week.
2. Listen to your body.
3. Try to work out for a minimum of fifteen minutes and gradually increase your time as you get in better shape.

Before the actual activity, warm up by performing a lower-intensity exercise to gradually prepare the body for greater movement. For instance, if you're going to jog around a track, walk a lap first. This gradual increase in exercise intensity allows adequate blood flow to the heart and muscles to prevent damage to the muscles and heart. Include static stretching in the warm-up to increase flexibility or improve range of motion, allowing you to move more freely. This prevents injury due to tight, stiff muscles. If you are going to swim, instead of focusing on the lower body, stretch the upper body (arms, shoulders, back, and chest). Stretching can be performed to a greater degree after the workout, when the muscles are really warm.

You should not feel any pain, only mild tension from the stretch. Hold the stretch for at least ten to thirty seconds. Finally, you need to include a cooldown at the end of your workout. The warm-up prepares the body to increase its activity; the cooldown prepares the body to decrease the activity before you actually stop. Its major purpose is to prevent a major drop in arterial blood pressure, which can cause an insufficient supply of blood to reach the brain and cause dizziness, light-headedness, and even fainting.

Whatever physical activity you decide to do, it is important to first consult your physician, start out slowly, and set small, realistic goals.

As I mentioned earlier, physical principles are used to describe spiritual principles throughout the Bible. Jesus taught with parables, using agricultural jobs and other activities the people could relate to, to explain the things of God. Paul does the same in many of his writings. In many instances in the Bible he compares the Christian life to a "race" or athletic competition. The Christian life is often called the Christian "walk" as well.

In I Corinthians, Chapter 9, verses 24–27, Paul uses the illustration of preparing for athletic competitions to explain the attitude one should have about the Christian life. Athletic competitions or games were prevalent in biblical days, and people took pride in preparing for them. They prepared with one purpose in mind—to achieve their goal so they could win the prize. Obtaining their goal required discipline and order in their lives. They watched their food intake and physically trained their bodies. They prepared with strengthening and endurance activities and also exercises that improved their agility. They understood that it takes time and commitment.

Paul describes running and boxing competitions. In a race and in a boxing match, there is only one victor. During Paul's time the winner of these contests was crowned with a wreath. In these verses of Corinthians, Paul compares living a Christian life to preparing for an athletic competition.

People should live with a purpose in mind: obtaining the prize. The athlete's prize was a perishable crown. As a Christian, all who are prepared will win an imperishable crown and life in eternity with God. This principle can apply in every area in your life. Achieving a goal, physically or spiritually, is going to require discipline, training, commitment, and order in your life.

To do well in college, you study and prepare for exams. You can't hang out every night and party and live a life full of disorder and chaos if you want to achieve your goal. If you want to be a success-ful Christian, you prepare by setting aside time for prayer, Bible study, and worship. Losing weight and keeping it off requires the same type of attitude. Start out with a purpose in mind and keep your eyes focused on the goal. Not only is the goal to get the physi-cal results you want, but it is also to gain spiritually. As you improve your health and feel better, you will be able to be everything that God wants you to be. He will be able to use you to encourage and help others because of your personal accomplishments.

Remember: Keep your eyes on the prize.

Weight resistance activities are important because they increase lean body mass (shaping, defining, and toning the body), decrease the risk of bone loss, and increase metabolism, which helps you lose more body fat.

Because of the subsequent improvement of the musculoskeletal system, strength training is recommended to help us perform the activities of everyday life and decrease the risk of injury. Weight re-sistance activities include working out with weights at the gym or at home, with dumbbells, or with weight resistance bands or tubes. Some people are creative, using books, pans, and soup cans to help strengthen their muscles.

After I lost a significant amount of weight, my skin was not as tight and toned as it was before I gained the weight. I had to work with weights to get back in shape. I still do not like working out but I like a firm, toned body; therefore, I have dumbbells and weight resistance bands at home and I use them, performing toning activities at least twice a week. Contrary to what you have heard, you will not get big and bulky if you exercise with weights. Women do not have enough testosterone, the male hormone that causes the growth in muscle tissue, to look like Hercules.

Another myth is that you must lose weight first, then start toning. The truth is, toning your body will help you lose weight faster than just doing aerobics alone. As you increase your muscle tissue, you increase your metabolism, the rate at which your body burns energy. Muscle needs more fuel than fat does; muscle burns more calories.

Muscle tissue also weighs more than fat. So when you start toning your body, do not be alarmed if the scale does not show a weight loss. You may notice the change in your clothes before you actually see a change in the scale.

Many people allow the scale to control them. Try to stay away from the scale. Weigh yourself weekly or monthly, but not every day. Remember, it takes time. It took time to develop bad habits and to get out of shape; it will take time and commitment to develop good health habits and get in shape. Most people give up because they don't see results fast enough. I told you before: Don't focus on your body, just do what it takes, and don't be surprised when others notice the change first.

Although I am a fitness trainer, like many of you, due to my lifestyle, job, and family responsibilities, I don't have time to go to the gym or work out all the time. But my workout plan of doing aerobic activities at least three days a week for at least twenty to forty-five minutes and toning at least twice a week helps me maintain a healthy body. My health is important to me.

I admit that at one time I felt bad that I was an aerobics instructor who was not a size 2 or 3. But I have accepted my body type and the fact that I am short, compact, and thick in certain areas. As long as I can perform many or most activities with ease and without fatigue and I do not have a lot of body fat, I am really fine with my body. God did not make me thin, but He wants me healthy. I have accepted His beautiful creation. My body will never have control over me again. I thank God for deliverance.

Balance your activity with your caloric intake

It's really a shame that health and fitness have become so complicated. It really should not be so hard to lose weight. If you are journaling now, as you should be, you have a realistic idea of your eating habits. I mentioned earlier that many people say they don't know why they are gaining weight or can't lose it, but when they actually write down everything they eat, drink, or snack on, they are surprised by how many calories they consume daily. I also mentioned balance in the very beginning of this chapter. This is what weight loss and weight management are all about. It is a balancing act.

The Book of Leviticus is like a manual, or how-to guide, that explains the duties of the priest and the people. It also contains regulations and states the standards that God instructed Moses to give to the people. In Chapter 19, God issues a number of moral directives and commands in the people's dealings. Leviticus 19:36 reads, *"You shall have honest scales, honest weights, an honest ephah, and an honest hin: I am the Lord your God, who bought you out of the land of Egypt."*

God was instructing the people to use honest scales and honest weights. In the early days there was not a standard of weighing and measuring, and some vendors unfairly weighted their scales so that items cost more when they sold them and the vendors gained greater profits. As part of God's moral standards for the people, He forbade them to participate in this dishonest practice. He wanted their measurements and balances to be honest.

If they didn't use proper balances, the dishonest gained more money but faced God's punishment. When we cheat ourselves when it comes to the energy balance equation, not only do we gain weight but we also put ourselves at risk for other illnesses and diseases. We use the heavy scale of all those extra calories and little activity, and then wonder where all those extra pounds came from. We want to be light, yet we eat lots of heavy foods. When you compare what you eat to your energy expenditure or activity level, what do you get? Are you truly honest with yourself? Think about the foods you consume daily. Your snacks. How about your exercises? Just like there were certain consequences for the people who used dishonest scales, there are consequences when there is no balance to your eating and exercise habits. And we have a system to determine food weight and calories: labels.

Look at this very realistic example: If I am maintaining my weight and then all of a sudden I add a candy bar and some cookies to my daily diet, these extra calories eventually produce a weight gain, especially if I don't increase my physical activity. For every extra 3,500 calories consumed and not burned off, I gain one pound. If the extra candy bar and cookies increase my calorie intake to 3,500 calories extra a week, I gain one pound per week. Imagine how much I gain in a year. When I think about this, I understand how I gained so much weight in the past.

If you are really honest with yourself, can you admit that you usually know when you overdo it? Even before you kept a journal, didn't you know when you ate until your stomach was full and bloated or when you ate a lot of fattening, fried, or sugary foods and snacks? Or do you remember going back for a second or even a third serving or plate?

It is very simple. If you overeat or eat foods high in calories, then overweight will be the outcome. Don't overeat and you won't be overweight. If you exercise and burn more calories than you eat, then weight reduction is the result. If you want to maintain your weight, then you need to consume around the same amount of energy that you use. Balance is the key, and I'm going to help you develop or maintain this balance. Here are some tips:

DON'T EAT MORE THAN YOU'RE WILLING TO WORK OFF

If you know you are not an active person or do not have a job requiring a lot of physical exertion, why eat like you do? Many people fill their plates to the rim, go back for seconds after sitting in the office all day at the computer, and then wonder why they gain weight. If you don't want to gain the extra pounds, don't eat like you do. If you are trying to maintain your weight and decide to enjoy some of your favorite foods high in calories, just pick up your activity level to burn off the extra calories. Remember, extra calories, extra fat.

EAT THE MAJORITY OF YOUR CALORIES DURING THE DAY WHEN YOU ARE MOST ACTIVE

This is where many of us make our biggest mistake with food. For years dinner was always considered the most important and largest meal. Although dinner is very important because it is the time for the family to get together, it is the mealtime that can truly add on the pounds. Most people are typically more active during the day because that's the time they're out working and doing other activities. By the time they come home in the evening from work, they are winding down and starting to prepare for bed. You should eat fewer calories at dinner because your body requires fewer calories at that hour.

Ideally, breakfast should be your largest meal because you need the energy to start a brand-new day. If you can't eat a large breakfast or if you're not hungry, think about why. At one time I wasn't hungry in the mornings, either. Then I learned that the reason I wasn't hungry was that I ate a heavy dinner or I ate late at night. I guarantee that if you eat a light dinner, you wake up ready to eat breakfast first thing, or as soon as you get in to work. Just look at the word: break-fast. The morning meal is so important because you are breaking your fast, those hours when you weren't eating.

I also discovered why I woke up so sluggish and drowsy many mornings. Overeating taxes the body at night, causing it to work to digest the food while you are sleeping. Therefore, late-night eating or eating a heavy dinner caused me to wake up tired, irritable, and sluggish. Don't go to sleep on a full stomach. Don't eat dinner later than 7 P.M.—always at least a few hours before you go to bed.

If you get hungry later in the evening, fruit is a better choice for a late snack. Don't go to bed absolutely hungry. You should feel like you could eat something if you wanted to.

Although it is recommended that breakfast be the heaviest meal, I cannot eat a heavy breakfast, so my lunch is generally my largest meal. By lunchtime I am ready for some *real food.* My lunch is what most people consider dinner. I try to keep my actual dinner light, with maybe a small portion of meat, some vegetables, and fruit for dessert.

Most people are tired after they eat because they either overeat or eat foods high in fats, which make them feel tired. A light meal low in fat will not affect you this way. Remember also, if you eat late or eat a heavy dinner, you are sleeping on all those extra calories, and extra calories mean extra fat.

Set aside a specific time to exercise

It seems that if you ask most people why they don't exercise, when they know it's good for their health, they say, "I don't have the time." If we are honest with ourselves we realize we make the time to do anything else we want to do or consider important, but when it comes to our health, there is always something else we need to do that's more important. Many women, specifically, take the time to go to the beauty parlor religiously to keep their hair looking nice, get their nails done, and even get a pedicure. We find time to talk to our girlfriends on the phone for hours and watch the soaps and other television programs. But if we don't take the time to take care of our health, we won't be around long enough to enjoy the many blessings waiting for us.

Although I am glad that my father is no longer suffering, I really miss him and often wish he were still around. I don't know how long I am going to live, but when I saw the effect that neglecting my body had on the outside and the way it made me feel (tired, sluggish, irritable, depressed, etc.), I could only imagine what was going on inside. I decided I was going to be healthy, and just like King David said in Psalm 118:17, *"I shall not die, but live, and declare the good works of the Lord."* I want to be around a long time for my children and through the help of God live to help others who struggled with the problems I had.

As a single mother of three, for many years I really didn't have the time to exercise. But it was up to me to make it a priority in my life. I still don't have time to exercise. I make time. I'm the typical American who has to work to live and provide for my family. And although I am a personal trainer, I do not spend one to two hours in the gym every day. In addition to fulfilling ministerial responsibilities, attending church services and meetings, and teaching workshops and seminars, I have to work, train clients, and take care of my family—which includes cooking, washing, cleaning the house, and helping with homework. I also have to drive three daughters to their various activities. Sometimes I don't know if I am coming or going. But I can tell you one thing: If I didn't make the time to exercise, I wouldn't be able to do what God has created for me to do at this point in my life.

I discovered that the healthier I am, the more I am able to do. Studies show that just losing five pounds can help you feel better. If you don't believe it, put on five-pound ankle weights. Walk around in them for a substantial period of time, then take them off and notice how light you feel in comparison to when you were walking around with the extra five pounds.

One thing I learned when it comes to exercise is that you need to set aside a specific time and stick to it so that it becomes a part of your life. The next thing I learned is when it's time to exercise, you can't think about it; you have to just do it. If you think too hard, you'll talk yourself out of it. Once you do it over and over, it becomes a habit and you'll feel strange, as if something is missing, when you don't exercise.

As a mother, especially when my kids were younger, my time to exercise was first thing in the morning. If I did not exercise before I went to work, I did not have the chance to do it once I came home because I had to cook and take care of my young children. Even though my children are older, this is still the best time for me because so many other things seem to come up during the day. Sometimes you must sacrifice and wake up twenty or thirty minutes earlier, but it will be worth it in the long run.

In the beginning, as your body is adjusting, you may feel a little tired. After a while you wake up more easily and feel strange if you don't get up and move. You can jog, ride a stationary bike, or walk on a treadmill early in the morning. Going to the gym is always an option, too. I didn't want to go to the gym because in the time it took for me to drive there and back, I could finish my entire exercise routine at home.

There are many options, such as using your lunch hour on the job to work out, go for a walk outside, or walk around in the building. Many companies now have workout facilities available for their employees. Perhaps you can exercise before it's time to start working, during part of your lunch hour, or before you go home.

Working out in the evenings is perfect for some people as well. They look forward to burning off the stress from the day. You can also work out on stationary equipment while talking on the phone or watching TV at home. It is all about prioritizing. If you really want to do it, you can make the time.

During the fourth day of creation, God ordered the universe so that He could give us time. He gave us twenty-four hours in a day, seven days in a week, approximately thirty days in a month, and 365 days in a year. Just as we are to be good stewards over our bodies, which belong to God, we are also to be good stewards over the time God has given us. How much time do you spend on the telephone? Watching TV? Or even eating or going out? Where and with whom do you spend most of your time? What do you spend most of your time doing? Prioritizing your time to make the most use out of it is very important. The Book of Ecclesiastes says there's a time for everything, and Ephesians 5:15–16 reads, *"See then that you walk circumspectly, not as fools, but as wise, redeeming the time, because the days are evil."*

God wants us to walk circumspectly by doing things the right way. He does not want us to behave foolishly and neglect those things that are really important. This world tells us that obtaining power, money, and status is important, but doing the things of God is what will last forever. God wants us to use wisdom in everything we do. Is it wise to neglect your health and not expect to eventually get ill? God also wants us to make the most out of every opportunity, "redeeming the time." If you have to talk on the phone or watch your favorite television program, get a stationary bike or treadmill and go for it.

When I think of time and stewardship, I think about a parable that Jesus told. In the parable of the talents (Matthew 25:14–30), Jesus tells a story about a man traveling to a far country. Before the man left, he gave talents to his servants. To one servant he gave five talents of money, to another two talents, and to another one talent, each according to his own ability. Then he left on his journey.

The servant who received five talents made five more talents and the servant who received two gained two more talents. But the servant who was given the one dug in the ground and hid his lord's money. After a long time the lord came back to settle accounts with the servants. So the one who had received five talents brought five additional talents to his lord, the one who received two brought him the two additional talents, and the lord said to both servants, "Well done, good and faithful servant; you were faithful over a few things, I will make you ruler over many things. Enter into the joy of your lord." Then the servant who had received one talent told his lord he was afraid and so he hid the talent in the ground. But his lord answered and said to him, "*You wicked and lazy servant . . . , you ought to have deposited my money with the bankers, and at my coming I would have received back my own with interest.*"

This seems like a harsh comment, but it wasn't at all. The master gave each servant a talent according to his own ability, so no one received more than he could handle. While the first two servants acted wisely and made the most of the talents, the last servant was lazy and selfish. Likewise, God gives us time, money, gifts, talents, children, jobs, and other blessings that He expects us to use wisely.

We are not owners of anything, not even our time. We are only caretakers. Although the first servant doubled his five talents and the second servant doubled his two, God was just as pleased with both of them and gave them the same response. So the issue as demonstrated in this parable is not how much you have but how well you use what you have.

I know there are many exercise programs claiming to be "the one" to get you in shape. Whatever you do, get your body moving. Find something you sincerely like, something you can stick to. If you do not enjoy the activity, it will probably soon become work and you will find yourself in a slump again.

There may be some activities you've never considered. Look at the following list and choose those activities you find exciting: aerobics (including cardio-kickboxing, cycling, hi-low aerobics, step aer-

obics, water aerobics, etc.), badminton, baseball, basketball, bicy-
cling, body shaping (with light dumbbells, resistance bands, or
tubes), bowling, canoeing, dance, golf, gymnastics, hiking, hockey,
horseback riding, ice skating, jogging, jumping rope, karate, kayak-
ing, martial arts, racquetball, inline skating, roller skating, rowing,
running, skiing, softball, stationary equipment (such as bike, rower,
and treadmill), swimming, tennis, volleyball, walking, water skiing,
yoga, Pilates, and weight training.

PRAYER

Say this prayer and write it on a card so you can keep it with you
and read it when you need encouragement:

Dear God,
I know that I have neglected my body by allowing other things in
my life to have priority over my health. I have not taken the time
to exercise, which is good for my health and my overall well-
being. You are a God of order and a God of action. Exercise helps
keep my body in order and functioning properly. The Bible tells
me in Proverbs 19:15 that laziness casts one into a deep sleep. I
want to be vibrant and more energetic so I can do all of my daily
activities more easily. Taking care of my health is pleasing you be-
cause your desire is for me to prosper in all things and to be in
good health, just as my soul prospers (III John, verse 2). I am ad-
mitting right now that I need your help. I need you to strengthen
me, encourage me, and lead me to do what is right. I am going
to take a step of faith and set aside the time to get up and start
moving. I believe once I take the first step you will be right there
to help me to continue. Please help me stay focused on achieving
my health goals. I thank you right now for the wonderful changes

that are going to take place in my life because I am taking the time to care for my body. Amen.

Study Scriptures

III JOHN, VERSE 2
Beloved, I pray that you may prosper in all things and be in health, just as your soul prospers.

Ephesians 5:15–16
See then that you walk circumspectly, not as fools but as wise, redeeming the time, because the days are evil.

ACTIVITIES

1. Walk up the stairs instead of using the elevator.

2. Park your car at the far end of the lot and walk briskly to your destination.

3. Put on some of your favorite Christian music and clean your house with gusto.

4. If you sit at work at a computer most of the day, get up and take five-minute breaks, stretching and walking.

5. Walk your dog, or walk around your neighborhood or to the park with family members after dinner.

6. Walk around your building during your lunch break, walk around the mall, or start a walking group on your job, in your church, or in your community.

7. Wash your car, mow your lawn, or do some gardening.

8. Play actively with your kids. Jump rope, play kickball, volleyball; skate, go inline skating, bowl.

9. When you have to use the restroom at work, walk to one farther away from your office.

10. Put on some of your favorite Christian music and just move. Do jumping jacks, jog in place, step side to side. Just have a great time glorifying God by taking care of his temple.

11. Keep an exercise log or journal. Write in your journal or keep a separate log for your exercise schedule and stick to it. Write your schedule activities for the week and check what you actually do. Write down what activity you plan to do and on what days. For instance, if you plan to include three days of aerobics and two days of toning, then Monday, Wednesday, and Friday could be the days you plan to walk for thirty minutes and Tuesdays and Thursdays could be your days for toning. Just remember, the muscles need rest. You wouldn't do the toning days back-to-back if you were toning the same muscle groups. Also include variety in your activities to avoid getting bored. Change the activities or switch the days you do certain activities. As you start to put it all together and you look at your food journal, your exercise log, and your body, it will become clear what it takes to get the results you want. You will see whether overeating is the problem or whether it's the lack of activity, and you can make the necessary adjustments.

12. Get familiar with your body. Look in the mirror and take a real good look at your body. If you don't like your physical condition, love yourself knowing that you are still beautiful in the sight of God. If the only way you feel you will love yourself is if you are smaller, your body size is not the only problem. Don't place your value on your body size or body parts. This was very difficult for me because I compared myself to what I looked like before I had children. Even as I started losing weight, I was so self-critical I couldn't enjoy the compliments people gave me. I still remembered the young, athletic girl who had a twenty-three-inch waistline, not one inch of fat, and a tight, firm body. I was fighting a no-win battle. I had to accept a new body and how it had changed due to childbearing. I had to concentrate on making it healthier instead of reaching for someone

else's goals or the body I used to have. I had to also look at myself with new eyes informed by the truth.

For instance, I didn't like the way my breasts looked after childbirth. But I had to look at the reality. Just as society emphasizes long, slender, size 4 models in magazines, it has also overrated breasts. When we have children and as we get older, real breasts simply do not stand at attention and remain as firm as grapefruits. For the most part, breasts were created to feed babies, and when they serve their purpose or as gravity takes over with age, our breasts seem to relax. I had to accept this and get on with the business of taking care of my health.

If you find yourself stuck on one body feature, learn how to appreciate the whole self, not just the body. The essence of who you are is not wrapped up in your body or a body part.

In I Samuel, Chapter 16, God instructed the prophet Samuel to go and anoint the next king over Israel. At the time Saul was legally the king. He was tall, handsome, and impressive-looking. Although he was a good-looking man, he was disobedient to God and his heart wasn't right. God didn't want Samuel to make the same mistake that the people had made with Saul, so when God sent him out to anoint the next king, He told him in verse 7, *"Do not look at his appearance or at his physical stature because I have refused him. For the Lord does not see as man sees; for man looks at the outward appearance, but the Lord looks at the heart."*

Samuel initially anointed the sons of Jesse who looked like kings (in his eyes), but none of them were chosen by God. God had chosen David, the youngest of Jesse's sons, to be the next king over Israel. David may not have looked like a king, but God had chosen him because of his sincere heart. The word "heart" in this text refers to the inner person, the real self. When we look at people's appearance alone, we miss wonderful attributes or qualities in people who do not have the physical attributes we find attractive. And if we are concerned only about our outward appearance, we never take the time to develop the real person, the inner self. God doesn't even judge us by our outward appearance; He judges a person's character.

Focus on the positive attributes God has given you. The devil uses society's obsession with so-called physical perfection to keep us in bondage so we cannot enjoy the absolute freedom, peace, and joy God has made available to each of us. If the Bible tells me I was made in the image of God and I was fearfully and wonderfully made and I can have an abundant life and peace of mind right here on earth, that's worth praising and thanking God for even as I continue to strive to be all that He has created me to be.

Now take a second look at your body. This time use your imagination a little. Imagine if the fat pockets or extra rolls were gone. Imagine if your waistline was trimmer and your stomach was flatter and tighter. Imagine if your buttocks, legs, and thighs were firmer and shapelier. Imagine if those wings in the back of your arms were gone. Imagine if you stood more erect with an improved and more confident posture. Imagine if your breasts appeared to be more lifted and firmer because of stronger, tighter muscles, which support the breast.

Well, I am a witness that some or all of this is possible with a little commitment and work. The problem with many of us is, we want these results, but we don't want to work for them. You do not have to go to the gym and train like a bodybuilder or a marathon runner to get good results, but you do have to get moving and stick to it. Most people never get to see these results because they give up too soon. Even if genetics stop you from getting the results you desire, you will look significantly better by shaping up what you have.

In this book, especially because it is a "spiritual" book, I could tell you not to worry about how you look because it really isn't important, but that is not reality. Although society overrates physical appearance, it is okay to care about how you look. Yet your appearance should not determine your self-worth. Our physical appearance is only a small piece of the pie when it comes to the whole person. Someone can be breathtakingly beautiful on the outside and mean and ugly on the inside. Or they can be unattractive on the outside and one of the most beautiful people you will ever meet. So although you want to look a certain way, don't focus on your body. Ultimately you need to love yourself and accept your body no matter what it looks like. Once you accept it and move on, you can "strive to be fit and the look will be your tip." Focus on just doing the activities and stop looking in the mirror constantly or weighing yourself every day.

I am a personal witness; if you stay consistent, good results are inevitable. And yes, in the beginning it requires some additional effort until your body gets used to your new activities and lifestyle. But you will not regret the effort. The Bible says in Hebrews, Chapter 11, that faith without works is dead. Many of us want to believe, but very few are willing to work. God doesn't want you to sit back and complain and constantly say what you need or want to do. He wants you to do something about it. As you begin to act by faith, just ask God to give you the strength, the desire, and the help you need to commit to taking care of your body, His temple. And remember, there is nothing wrong with wanting to look better, as long as your body doesn't become your primary focus or the "god" in your life.

When Trinity Broadcast Network called me to be the cohost of *TotaLee Fit* with Lee Haney, I questioned why God would allow them to call at that particular time in my life. I was in physical therapy and experiencing pain after having a second surgery on my leg. I couldn't exercise regularly and had gained about seven pounds.

I considered telling TBN no. My other choice was to lose weight the unhealthy way, by going on a very restrictive low-calorie diet.

But I knew that if I did this, it could possibly start an unhealthy cycle of fasting and bingeing. I would also be going against everything I believe.

I felt desperate, yet I heard a voice inside me telling me that it wasn't about the look. It was about being healthy and it was about being who I am to God. My mother told me the same thing, that people in the world might focus on the outside but what was really important to God was the person I was inside and the relationship I had with Him.

What really blessed me and motivated me to go on the show was when my mother gave me a card and wrote on it how proud she was of me and how blessed she was to have a child who truly loves God and has a desire to please Him and help others.

I had to let go of any vanity I possessed. Would I do His work being healthy and fit for Him, or would I allow the world's standards to cause me to lose focus of what was really important?

I thank God every time I am able to exercise without pain because there are some people who can't walk or stand. I thank God I am no longer in bondage to my body and that how I feel about myself is not based on my physical appearance or my "body parts," but on my relationship with God.

Get rid of the issues that stop you from being "fit for God"

1. LACK OF SELF-CONTROL
Self-control is a fruit of the Spirit of God. If you allow Him to lead you and have control over your life, He will give you the strength you need to say no. **Galatians 5:22–23** *But the fruit of the Spirit is love, joy, peace, longsuffering, kindness, goodness, faithfulness, gentleness, self-control. Against such there is no law.*

2. "I'M BIG-BONED LIKE EVERYONE IN MY FAMILY"
Many of your physical attributes and characteristics such as your

appearance, height, body structure, and even metabolism were determined by your genetics. Many eating habits also run in our families, but they don't come from our parents' genes. Most people learn how to eat and cook from their parents. If their parents cooked high-fat foods, then most likely they will grow up and do the same. What does this have to do with being "big-boned"? Nothing. But many women have offered this explanation to me as a reason for being overweight. When I looked at the eating habits of most of them and their families, everyone ate heartily and didn't exercise. Yes, many people are naturally large, but what's important is health. Many people who are in great shape are considered overweight according to the height and weight charts because muscle weighs more than fat. The American College of Sports Medicine defines obesity as the percentage of body fat that increases the risk for disease. Therefore a person can appear small or average in size and still be considered obese if they have a high body fat percentage. You can get a good idea of your body composition by getting a body fat analysis, available through health care professionals or fitness trainers. **Hebrews 12:1–2** *Therefore we also, since we are surrounded by so great of a cloud of witnesses, let us lay aside every weight, and the sin which so easily ensnares us, and let us run with endurance the race that is set before us looking unto Jesus, the author and finisher of our faith . . .*

3. "EXERCISE IS PAINFUL AND UNCOMFORTABLE"

For years we all have heard, "No pain, no gain." But exercise doesn't have to be painful in order to be effective. In fact, you shouldn't exercise until it hurts. Pain is a warning sign from the body. If you are in pain and very uncomfortable, that's a clear indication that your body is signaling you to stop. It's very important for each person to work out at his or her own fitness level. If you are a beginner, start out slowly. Moderate exercise is most effective for fat-burning; activity that causes total exhaustion is not. Work out gradually. As you improve your strength and fitness level, then you can increase your exercise intensity. It is possible that you will experience mild to moderate soreness as your muscles make the necessary adjustments to accommodate their new workload. Stretching before, during, and after exercising can help alleviate any muscle soreness and tightness that may occur. **Romans 12:1–2** *I beseech you therefore, brethren, by the mercies of God, that you present your bodies a living sacrifice, holy, acceptable to God, which is your reasonable service. And do not be conformed to this world, but be transformed by the renewing of your mind, that you may prove what is the good and acceptable and perfect will of God.*

4. "I DON'T WANT TO START EXERCISING BECAUSE IF I STOP THE MUSCLE WILL TURN INTO FAT"

When God said my people perish for lack of knowledge, He knew what He was talking about. I've heard many myths about fitness and working out over the years. Fat and muscle are two different types of body tissue. One cannot turn into the other. You can actually have fat on top of muscle, which also contributes to a larger appearance. A good example is dealing with the stomach. Many women, specifically, come to me wanting to lose their stomach. They ask me to show them exercises for their midsection. I show them the exercises, but I also stress that they have to lose body fat in order to lose the fat on top of the stomach—through fat-burning exercises and proper nutrition. Many of them don't take heed but instead do numerous crunches day and night. I've had some women tell me they do over a hundred crunches a night and their stomach looks even larger. They increased the muscle tissue but they didn't do any aerobic activities to burn fat and wound up with muscle underneath the fat. You cannot spot reduce. You cannot just work one area of your body and expect to lose fat in that area only. Cardiovascular activity such as walking, jogging, biking, and many others are great ways to burn fat. So the problem is not the muscle turning to fat; it's that if you consume more calories than you burn off, the extra calories are stored as fat. If you have a concern, don't accept myth as truth. Make sure you get the answer from a professional or from a reputable health book. **Proverbs 10:14** *Wise people store up knowledge, but the mouth of the foolish is near destruction.*

5. "I USED TO EXERCISE, BUT IT'S HARD TO GET STARTED AGAIN"

This is so true. It's hard to get started exercising if you have never done it before, and it's hard if you have stopped and have to get going again. The only thing I can really share is: You just have to do it. You have to stop saying what you need to do or what you are going to do and make it happen. Set aside a specific time that you are going to commit to exercising. When the time comes, don't debate whether or not to start on that day. When the thoughts of doubt enter your mind, immediately rebuke them. If you think too long you will talk yourself out of it (I know from experience), and if you keep making excuses you'll never get started. Even if you know it's the right thing to do and have the right intentions, it won't do you any good if you don't put your knowledge into practice. **James 1:22** *But be doers of the word and not hearers only, deceiving yourselves.*

6. SEEKING OTHER PRIORITIES

People seek more money, a better job, more education, and longer work hours all at the expense of their health. God wants us to be successful and prosper. However, if we put Him first, He'll take care of all these other things in our lives. **Matthew 6:33** *But seek first the kingdom of God and His righteousness, and all these things shall be added to you.*

Week Five
Trim the Fat

*. . . So God Created Great Sea Creatures and Every Living
Thing That Moves . . .*

—Genesis 1:21

As God was creating the earth and all that is in it, after each step He said, "It is good." He was delighted to see His accomplishments toward His final goal. Likewise, as you move toward your goal, step by step, God is delighted. It's like salvation; you don't become saved one day and perfect the next. The word of God tells us we have to work out our own soul salvation (Philippians 2:12). It is not an instantaneous occurrence. We don't improve in every area of our lives all at once. It is a step-by-step process of overcoming one area and then moving on to the next.

Consider again the order of God's work, how even in the making of animals there was a plan. Let's look at the fifth day of creation, starting at Genesis 1:20. *"Then God said, 'Let the waters abound with an abundance of living creatures, and let birds fly above the earth across the face of the firmament of heavens.'"* Genesis 1:20–23 states that God made all of the living creatures of the water and all of the winged birds and He blessed them, and said, *"Be fruitful and multiply, and fill the waters in the seas, and let birds multiply on the earth."* This means, when it comes to food, we now have our fish, chicken, and turkey.

On the sixth day, God created animals of the earth. Genesis 1:24 reads, *"Then God said, 'Let the earth bring forth the living creature according to its kind: cattle and creeping thing and beast of the earth, each according to its kind'; and it was so."* God has now made the other animals, including the beef and pork that many people eat.

Now look at the order in which God created animals. He created fish and chicken on the fifth day, then beef and pork on the sixth day. Tips on healthier living from various nutrition and health experts recommend eating more fish and chicken and less red meat (or animals from the earth) because they are higher in fat.

Why do you think health experts recommend this order? Because beef and pork generally have a higher fat and cholesterol content than chicken and fish, which can contribute to extra weight and the risk of illnesses.

Heart disease is the number one killer in America. According to the American Heart Association, eating a diet low in fat and cholesterol can reduce your risks for heart disease. A diet low in fat can also reduce your risk for high cholesterol, diabetes, certain cancers, and other illnesses, including premature physical deterioration.

Jessica was a client who came to me because she wanted to lose weight to feel comfortable in her bathing suit for her vacation in Hawaii. I wasn't surprised; many people initially come to me sparked by a special occasion. Some come to lose weight to get a higher rank in the military, some to look a certain way in their wedding dress or at their school reunion, and many to prepare for that summer swimwear.

Jessica said she had to lose weight fast because her vacation was coming up soon. She really did not care much for exercising, such as doing aerobics, jogging, or using weights, so I encouraged her to walk. She started walking daily with coworkers during her lunch break, and I worked with her twice a week for muscle toning. She began to notice a definite difference, but of course, the weight loss was not fast enough for her. She said she didn't eat much. When she started recording all the food she ate daily in her journal, we discovered it was true that she did not eat much, but the problem was that the food she ate was high in calories and fat.

The only thing she really had to do was to de-fat her foods, or reduce her intake of high-calorie foods. She did not overeat and she didn't eat late at night. But she ate fried foods regularly, and high-calorie baked goods and snacks. She ate salads and vegetables often, yet she loaded her salads with high-calorie, fattening salad dressing and she cooked her vegetables with pork. She also ate fried chicken most days of the week. As a matter of fact, she said she fried foods in her house almost every day or prepared a dish requiring beef or pork.

After looking at her journal, in addition to her walking and toning, she reduced her intake of fried foods and other high-calorie foods. The extra weight seemed to melt away. As her fitness trainer, I was absolutely amazed with her weight loss and physical improvement. She initially wanted to lose weight only for her vacation, but when she saw the results and realized the role that high-calorie or high-fat foods played in her health and that of her family, she continued cooking and eating healthier. Not only did Jessica achieve most of her weight loss goals for her vacation, but she also learned healthier habits that were a benefit for her and her loved ones for a lifetime.

At one time I counted and accounted for every calorie I ate. However, this kept me in bondage to food, worried about whether I could eat this food or that food. Although counting calories may help some people keep track of their food intake, you do not have to count calories if you put certain tips into practice. If you reduce your intake of high-calorie and fattening foods, you will eliminate most of the extra fat and calories in your diet that is stored as extra fat on your body. I do not count calories and I don't weigh my food to lose weight. When I did, I constantly missed my goal.

Let's look again at the Food Pyramid Guide that I first mentioned in Week Three (eating natural foods). Building a healthy body can be looked at like building a house. You must build a strong foundation if that house is going to stand. The Food Pyramid Guide helps you build that foundation.

If you look at the food groups in the pyramid from the bottom up, they are practically listed in the order in which God created them (although the milk group is listed before the meat group; most milk and cheese products all come from meat or animals).

MILK, YOGURT, AND CHEESE GROUP

Foods from the milk group are our body's best sources of calcium, an important mineral responsible for strong bones and teeth. Sufficient calcium is needed to prevent osteoporosis, a condition that causes the bones to easily fracture due to loss of bone density. Food included in this group, in addition to milk: ice cream, buttermilk, cottage cheese, frozen yogurt, shakes, and puddings. Without dairy products it would be hard to get enough calcium to keep the bones strong. Women, especially, often neglect the milk group; therefore, it is recommended that some of them take calcium supplements. But remember that vitamins and minerals are better absorbed when they are consumed in food sources. Some dairy products and other beverages and foods are now fortified with calcium.

The milk group is also a good source of vitamin A and vitamin D, phosphorous, potassium, protein, and riboflavin. The number of recommended daily servings for the milk group is two to three. The following serving sizes are according to the American Dietetic Association:

- 1 cup milk or buttermilk
- 1 cup yogurt
- $\frac{1}{2}$ cup evaporated milk

- $\frac{1}{3}$ cup dry milk
- $1\frac{1}{2}$ ounces natural cheese (Cheddar, mozzarella, Swiss, Monterey Jack)
- $\frac{1}{2}$ cup ricotta cheese
- 2 ounces processed cheese (American)
- $\frac{1}{2}$ cup frozen yogurt or 1 cup cottage cheese counts as $\frac{1}{2}$ serving; $\frac{1}{2}$ cup ice cream counts as $\frac{1}{3}$ serving

MEAT, POULTRY, FISH, DRY BEANS, EGGS, AND NUTS GROUP

Meats or animals make up most of this group. Man was initially a vegetarian because God first told man that he had all the vegetation from the earth to eat as food. Then after the flood during Noah's day, God said in Genesis 9:3, *"Every moving thing that lives shall be food for you. I have given you all things, even as the green herbs."* It is as though He is saying, "In addition to the vegetation I gave you to eat, you can also eat the meat of the animals." He continues to say in verse 4 that man shall not eat flesh with its life, that is, its blood (the blood of animals was to be drained before they were eaten).

I Timothy 4:4–5 reads, *"For every creature of God is good, and nothing is to be refused if it is received with thanksgiving; for it is sanctified by the word of God and prayer."* In this Scripture, Paul was commenting on the teachings of false teachers who came into the church. They gave stringent rules that forbade people to eat certain food. But Paul affirmed that everything God created is good and we should receive it with thanksgiving and prayer.

So eating meat is not wrong and there are not any "bad foods." According to the Scripture, God gave us these foods as gifts or blessings. However, when we overeat or practice gluttony, we are abusing what God has made available for us.

In Matthew 15:11, Jesus spoke to the Pharisees about this issue of eating and drinking. The Pharisees were concerned with Jewish regulations about the manner in which foods were handled and the fact that certain foods could not be eaten because they were considered "unclean." What Jesus said about this matter offended the Pharisees. Christ said, *"Hear and understand: Not what goes into the mouth defiles a man; but what comes out of the mouth, this defiles a man."* He was saying it's not eating certain foods that make you unclean, but what's in your heart and what is spoken from your mouth.

This again shows that there are no "bad foods," but that what is important is how we use these foods. We must not neglect the blessings God has given us.

Whether to be a vegetarian or to eat meat is clearly a choice, and I am not going to debate that in this book. Good health is what is important. But I am definitely an animal lover, so I sympathize with people who are disturbed when they hear cruel stories of how some animals are treated and killed for food. If you choose not to eat meat for whatever reason, make sure you eat a variety of plant foods to ensure you are getting sufficient nutrients for health.

So what is important about meat? As mentioned in Week Three, meat contains one of the essential nutrients: protein. Generally, animal products are the best sources of protein because they contain complete proteins (those with all of the essential amino acids). Animal products such as meat, eggs, cheese, milk, and yogurt contain a higher quality of protein than other foods do. Remember: Protein is the building material for the body. It makes up all the different tissues of the body (including muscle tissue) and it's needed for proper functioning of the body.

In addition to being the best source of protein, meats are the best sources of the iron called heme iron (for healthy blood), which is better absorbed by the body than the iron from plant food sources. Meat also supplies the body with B vitamins (vitamin B6, vitamin B12, thiamine, and niacin) and zinc.

Getting sufficient protein is also important for satiety and to prevent hunger. If your diet consists of mostly carbohydrates and sugars, you will never feel satisfied. But protein foods such as meat, eggs, and cheese satisfy the appetite. One of the reasons could be that protein foods take longer to digest.

If I eat only a bowl of cereal in the morning for breakfast, by lunch I am so hungry I may overeat. But if I also include eggs with my breakfast, I can hold out a little longer without feeling famished. Even at dinnertime, eating a piece of meat such as a salmon fillet or a chicken breast with a salad or vegetable is very satisfying, nutritious, and great for weight management.

The meat group on the pyramid includes a variety of foods: beef, chicken, turkey, pork, fish, game, eggs, dry beans, tofu, nuts, and peanut butter. Although dry beans, tofu, nuts, and peanut butter are actually plant foods, they are listed in this section of the pyramid because of their nutrient content. For instance, dry beans combined with grain (such as rice) make a complete protein. Beans are also an excellent source of complex carbohydrates and dietary fiber and should be included in the diet weekly. Dry beans are almost fat-free, but nuts and peanut butter are higher in fat and calories, so you need to go easy on these.

You can eat:

- 2 to 3 ounces cooked lean meat, poultry, or fish (4 ounces raw meat, poultry, or fish equal 3 ounces when cooked)
- 2 to 3 ounces lean sliced deli meat (turkey, ham, beef, or bologna)
- 2 to 3 ounces canned tuna or salmon, packed in water

. . . for a total of 5 to 7 ounces each day.

Count as 1 ounce of meat:

- ½ cup cooked lentils, peas, or dry beans
- 1 egg

- ¼ cup egg substitute
- 2 tablespoons peanut butter
- 4 ounces tofu

Count as 2 ounces of meat:

- ½ cup tuna or ground beef
- 1 small chicken leg or thigh
- 2 slices sandwich-size meat

Count as 3 ounces of meat:

- 1 medium pork chop
- ¼ pound hamburger patty
- 1 chicken breast
- 1 unbreaded, 3-ounce fish fillet
- cooked meat the size of a deck of cards

FAT, OILS, AND SWEETS

This is the tip of the pyramid, meaning these are the foods that we need to eat sparingly. They include butter, margarine, cream, cream cheese, oil, salad dressing, gravy, soft drinks, fruit drinks, jams, jellies, gelatin desserts, sugar, and candies. No recommended serving sizes are given to this group.

Even when I finally learned how to eat healthier, I still didn't have complete control over eating the foods in the fat, oils, and sweets group. In public or at work, I ate my healthy meals. People always commented and said, "La Vita always eats healthy." I felt so guilty because as I was lifting the fork to put salad in my mouth, I was creating my next meal in my mind. I couldn't wait to get home, where I could pig out. Whether I was typing on the computer, driving in

my car, or sitting in church during service—whatever I was doing—
I was thinking about my next high-fat, high-calorie meal. At any
given time I had an ongoing love relationship with three men: my
husband or boyfriend and the ice cream moguls Ben and Jerry. I was
addicted to food. It was exciting to think about my next meal and
snack. I ate snacks after I ate my meals. That's why it was so easy to
eat thousands of calories at any one time. I lived for the taste of fat
and sugar. I felt bad about myself, I felt bad about my life, and then
I had the negative words constantly spoken by my abuser.

Although physical abuse is very harmful and can be deadly, I feel
that mental and verbal abuse can be just as fatal. Physical abuse
harms the body, but verbal abuse kills the spirit. Physical wounds
take days or weeks to heal, but emotional wounds take even longer,
maybe even a lifetime to heal.

I mentioned earlier that according to the Bible, life and death are
in the power of the tongue. This means that what is spoken can be
life-supporting or deadly. I heard many words of death. But the food
made me feel alive: Pizza with plenty of cheese, Kentucky Fried
Chicken with biscuits, double cheeseburgers, french fries with
plenty of ketchup, steak sandwiches with cheese, and fried-fish
subs were just a few of my favorites. Late at night I prepared buttermilk pancakes, fried potatoes, and bacon and eggs with plenty of
cheese. This was definitely one of my favorite meals and I ate it anytime. I made my pancakes with only real buttermilk so they would
be smooth and tasty. Then I covered each pancake individually with
real butter and drowned them all in rich, thick King syrup. Shakes
were another favorite. I took ice cream and blended it in the blender
with whole milk, bananas, other fruits, or Hershey's chocolate syrup
and/or nutmeg, vanilla, and cinnamon. It was exciting to try different combinations. I knew that eating like this was unhealthy, but I
was out of control and the more I ate, the more I wanted to eat. I
knew that this was not God's desire for my life, but I couldn't stop.

I felt as though I needed the food for my satisfaction, the same way we need oxygen to sustain life.

When I think about high-fat foods, the story of Eli and his sons comes to mind. Eli was the high priest in Israel at Shiloh. He was the priest present when Hannah prayed to the Lord for a child. Although Eli had faith in God and was an excellent priest, he had trouble disciplining his two sons, Hophni and Phinebas. As priests, they took advantage of their positions and their father had difficulty enforcing their obedience to the Law.

In the Book of Leviticus, according to the Law, when people made sacrifices to the Lord, the priests were supposed to let the meat cook until all of the fat burned completely away. The fat, which adds flavor, was supposed to go up to the Lord as a sweet-smelling aroma. At times, Eli's sons ate the meat before the fat was burned completely off.

When God warned Eli (more than once) of the sin of his sons, Eli failed to correct them. Because Eli's sons were gluttonous eaters of meat and disobedient to God, God allowed them to be killed in battle by their enemy, and the Ark of the Covenant, which represented the presence of God, was taken from Israel. (The ark contained the two tablets of the Ten Commandments given to Moses by God.) When Eli heard this news, the Bible says, *"He fell off his seat backward, broke his neck and died, for he was old and heavy"* (I Samuel 4:18).

This story is symbolic of how gluttony and disobedience to God cause pain and death. The lesson is the same today. Research clearly shows that consuming foods high in fat increases your risk for disease and causes death.

Thank God that we are no longer under the Law in Leviticus or many of us would be dead because of our sin of eating the "fat." However, it is not realistic to say you want a fat-free diet. Fat is an essential nutrient needed by the body. The problem is, we consume more fat than the body actually needs, so it's stored on the body as extra weight.

The American Heart Association recommends eating a diet that derives no more than 30 percent of the total calories from fat. Here are some healthy tips for trimming the fat:

1. Make healthier meat selections (de-fat your meat)

- Eat more lean poultry, turkey, and fish (also, white meat poultry has less fat than dark meat).
- Remove the skin from poultry. Fat is found right under the skin, so by removing the skin you cut the fat in half.
- Choose lean cuts of meat. The words "round" and "loin" indicate leaner beef, and the words "loin" and "leg" indicate leaner pork or lamb. Avoid those meats that have a marbled appearance; they contain more fat (ask the butcher if in doubt).
- Trim all visible fat from meat. If you can see it, cut it off.
- Oven-fry chicken and fish. Fried chicken is twice as fattening as baked chicken. Dip in egg whites, coat with breadcrumbs, and bake on a nonstick pan (coated with vegetable spray).
- Bake, broil, roast, grill, oven-fry, stir-fry, sauté, or simmer meats.
- Limit your intake of processed meats such as hot dogs, bacon, and lunch meats. Many brands now have leaner, lower-fat selections.
- Drain off the oil or fat from meat after cooking it.
- Instead of using pork to season foods, cook these dishes with smoked turkey pieces.
- Replace ground beef with ground turkey or mix part lean ground beef (still drain off fat) in dishes such as spaghetti, lasagna, or chili.
- Select tuna packed in water instead of vegetable oil.

- Use 2 egg whites for 1 whole egg in recipes. The egg yolk contains the fat and cholesterol. Health experts recommend Americans eat no more than four yolks a week.

2. *Reduce your intake of high-fat dairy products*

- Switch from whole milk to low-fat milk or skim. Gradually reduce the fat content from 2 percent to 1 percent to skim. The fat content is the only difference.
- Try nonfat or low-fat versions of your favorite cheeses such as ricotta, and use skim-milk mozzarella.
- Buy sliced cheese so you can control portion sizes.
- Choose low-fat or skim buttermilk.
- Use evaporated, canned skim milk instead of cream or half-and-half.
- Try sherbet, frozen low-fat yogurt, ice milk, or frozen fruit bars instead of ice cream. (When buying some of these lower-fat versions, such as frozen yogurt, watch out for the calories. It may not have fat, but it can still be full of sugar and extra calories that still add extra fat on the body. Check the food label.)
- In recipes requiring milk, use skim milk instead of whole milk.
- Try a frozen fruit smoothie instead of a shake, or create your own using fruit, juice, skim milk, and/or low-fat yogurt.
- If you drink rice milk or soy milk, try the low-fat version.

3. *Limit your intake of foods high in fat, sugar, and sodium*

The tip of the pyramid includes foods that should be enjoyed in small amounts because they supply calories but few to no nutrients. These foods, as mentioned earlier, include fat, oils, and sweets. Although they are listed as part of the food pyramid, they are not considered a group because there is no minimum requirement or recommended serving sizes for them.

- Use margarine instead of butter, or try low-fat butter or margarine. Also whipped margarine or butter in tubs has less fat than the sticks.
- Go easy on the sour cream and cream cheese, or use low-fat varieties.
- Top pancakes, waffles, or French toast with fruit or fruit spread instead of syrup.
- Limit your salad dressing to 1 or 2 tablespoons, or use low-fat or fat-free.
- Limit your intake of fried foods (frying in oil can more than double the calories).
- When you go to restaurants, ask for your salad dressing or other fats on the side to control and limit the amount you use.
- Go easy on gravies, sauces, and spreads.
- Try fruit spreads on toast or bread instead of butter or margarine.
- Try herbs, spices, and lemon to flavor your meats instead of extra gravies, sauces, and fat drippings.
- Eat candy, pastries, pies, cake, and other sweets in moderation.
- Drink soft drinks in moderation. Drink more water and 100 percent fruit juices. (But watch your intake of juices because some of them have more calories than the actual fruit. Just one cup of orange juice may have 120 calories.)
- Replace sugary and fattening snacks and desserts with a variety of fresh fruits.
- Choose wholesome cereals that are low in sugar such as oatmeal or bran flakes. Avoid the high-fat cereals like granola or the sugary "kids'" cereals. Sprinkle granola in your yogurt or on top of other cereals for a nice crunch and treat.

- Eat a bagel for breakfast instead of a donut or pastries.
- Go easy on adding extra sugar to your foods. Try a variety of spices and fruit juices to add flavor to your food. For instance, instead of adding a lot of sugar to oatmeal, try cooking it with apple juice and cinnamon for a nice flavor, or try adding bananas or strawberries to dry cereal.

4. Shake the salt

Sodium is not listed at the tip of the pyramid, but many health experts suggest we limit our intake of foods high in salt.

Although many people use the terms "salt" and "sodium" interchangeably, there is a difference. The table salt that many people sprinkle on their food at home or in restaurants is "sodium chloride." Sodium chloride is composed of 40 percent sodium and 60 percent chloride.

Sodium is important because it controls the movement of fluids in and out of the body's cells, and it also regulates blood pressure, transmits nerve impulses, and helps the muscles, including the heart, to relax. Sodium is found naturally in foods; therefore, most people do not have a problem getting enough sodium. It's also added to many other foods we purchase, and many people add extra sodium from the saltshaker. In most healthy people, the kidney excretes extra sodium so that it is not stored in the body.

But research indicates there may be a link between sodium and high blood pressure in people who are considered "salt sensitive," or sensitive to the sodium that is in salt. It is estimated that up to 30 percent of America's population has high blood pressure that is sodium sensitive. For them, consuming too much sodium contributes to their blood pressure problems. High blood pressure or hypertension is a major risk factor for the number one killer in America: heart disease. High blood pressure also increases the risk for stroke and kidney disease.

There is no way to predict who may get high blood pressure due to sensitivity to sodium. However, health experts do know that

Americans have a much higher rate of high blood pressure than people in other countries and we also consume a lot more salt. Therefore, it is recommended that all Americans reduce their sodium intake. Again, make the changes gradually.

- Take the saltshaker off of the table. Use the out-of-sight, out-of-mind theory. Your taste buds will adjust to the natural taste of food in time.
- Season your foods with herbs, vinegar, lemon juice, fruit juices, and spices.
- Reduce your intake of high-salt foods such as chips, pretzels, popcorn, salted crackers, and salted nuts, or try the low-salt or unsalted versions.
- Don't add salt to the water when you cook pasta, rice, or vegetables.
- Nibble on fruits and vegetables rather than salty snacks.
- Limit your intake of prepared or processed foods, such as canned foods, boxed meals, canned soups, and frozen dinners, or choose the low-sodium versions.
- Reduce you intake of processed meats such as bologna, hot dogs, bacon, ham, sausage, pepperoni, and others high in sodium, or try the low-sodium versions.
- Go easy on condiments such as ketchup, mustard, relish, tartar sauce, soy sauce, and steak sauce.
- Check the Nutrition Facts panel on the food package for sodium content.

Remember: Do not eliminate all of your favorites at once. All foods, even the ones at the tip of the pyramid, can fit into a healthy lifestyle, but moderation is the key.

When you do decide to eat high-fat or high-calorie foods, just balance it out with your next meal and your activities. For instance, if you eat a high-fat breakfast that includes bacon or sausage and biscuits, have a lean turkey sandwich and a salad for lunch. If you eat a high-fat lunch of a cheeseburger and french fries, eat a light, low-fat dinner such as baked fish and a vegetable. And if you know you have consumed more calories than you normally do for the day, exercise a little longer that day.

As I have mentioned, the majority of my calories came from fats and sugar. I often ate over 2,000 calories' worth of cookies, ice cream, and cake at one sitting. It wasn't unusual for me to eat a whole row of Chips Ahoy chocolate chip cookies with a pint of ice cream. When I felt stuffed, I stopped and waited an hour or so until I no longer felt full, then I finished off the other row of cookies. Another favorite snack was sharp cheddar cheese and Ritz crackers. I ate eight ounces of cheese with a box of crackers at one sitting.

"I'll start my diet on Monday," I said repeatedly, as I ate what I promised myself would be my last large snack. One of the reasons I failed to lose weight was that I was trying to stop eating all of my favorite foods at the same time. This only set me up for bingeing. When I did taste the food again, I was out of control.

Let me share with you my twelve tips for avoiding temptation, overindulgence, or setbacks. I learned these tips through my own struggle with food and from my work with helping others. Use those that apply to you.

1. Don't deprive yourself of all your favorite foods. That would set you up for bingeing or overindulging. Enjoy your favorites *in moderation*. The problem is not the foods themselves, but how much of them you eat.

2. Choose a day of the week when you allow yourself to eat some of your favorites. I had to experiment to find out what works for me.

Normally I choose a weekend day. It gives me something to look forward to and helps me maintain a healthy diet during the week. Don't overindulge. Just enjoy one or a couple of your favorites.

My client Pamela eats two small chocolate cookies a day. This wouldn't work for me because two cookies would be a tease. Robyn, another client, eats high-fat breakfast meat such as bacon or sausage on Saturdays only, and has a slice of cake on Sunday after church.

3. Avoid the foods you don't have any control over. Although I am writing this book on health, and I am saved, sanctified, filled with the Spirit of God, and preaching the gospel of God, there are some foods that I just cannot eat a little of. Cheesecake is my challenge. I'm making myself hungry just writing about it.

One Sunday I wanted to support a friend at church. Her auxiliary was having a bake sale, so I bought a cheesecake, saying to myself, "I have control this time." But what did I do? I gave my three girls one slice each—and I ate the rest of the cake. I had to learn.

So the next time this friend was selling cheesecakes, I bought one, cut off a slice for me and one for each of my girls—and gave away the rest. I didn't take the extra home. As long as the cheesecake was in my presence, I was going to eat it.

You may have to change your behavior in other ways in order to stay away from certain foods. One client told me she had to avoid going into a certain bakery with her coworkers during lunch because she knew she would be out of control.

4. Don't bring certain foods home. If you know you don't have control over a particular food, don't bring it home. I had a client who bought pizzas to support a school fundraiser, and then gave them away. Another lady had to buy smaller birthday cakes for her children and give away the leftover slices in order to keep from eating them.

Be honest with yourself. Tell your spouse or family members what you are trying to do so they can support you.

5. Buy small sizes, not the extra-value bags or packs. You might get

more for your money by purchasing these larger packages; however, your health is more valuable than any amount of money you save. Also, don't snack out of a large bag. Place the snack in a plastic bag or a small bowl so that you can see exactly how much you're eating.

6. Recognize those people and places that influence you to overeat, and have a plan. By now you should have an idea of what triggers you to overeat (if you have been writing in your journal). Is it a girlfriend who always asks you to go out to eat with her? Ask her if you can try something different, like walking around a track or in the park. If you're going to the movies or to an event where there is food, eat before you leave home. When you eat at a restaurant, fill up on salad and vegetables so that you will be less likely to overeat. Prepare the family healthier meals and snacks also, but don't deprive them of some of their favorite snacks.

7. Deal with the emotional issue that may cause you to overeat. By recording in your journal you may find out you overeat when there is a lot of stress in your life; when you feel lonely or depressed; when you have problems on the job or in your home. As I mentioned earlier, I overate due to stress, anxiety, and depression. Now I know that as long as I live, there will always be stress. The only way I could deal with these emotional issues was to seek wisdom and knowledge from the word of God, and prayer. It's a daily process of renewing my mind and my strength through God's word. Through the Bible, I learned how to place my trust and confidence in God. I also found peace, hope, joy, love, and forgiveness for any situation. I discovered that God loved me dearly and I was not alone. The Bible has a word of encouragement for anything you may experience. To find a word for your particular reason, you can look in the concordance of your Bible or consider the reasons and excuses I list in each chapter.

8. Find a hobby or something productive to do. Many people I work with eat out of habit or boredom. Exercising, finding a hobby, or even volunteering can be the cure for boredom. Although we need to seek

the word of God for encouragement, there are still physical things that we can put into practice as we trust God to help us and guide us.

One client, who overate when she was bored, started planting flowers and became quite a gardener, which cured her boredom and made her appreciate God's creation. What are some of your interests? Do you like to help others? Do you enjoy working with your hands or with children? Maybe you can start a walking group in your neighborhood or volunteer at a nursing home or hospital.

9. Get out of the dieter's mind frame. The more you think about what you can't eat, the more you crave certain foods. When I got out of the dieter's mind frame of always being concerned about what I could and could not eat, to my surprise I stopped craving many high-calorie and fattening foods. As long as I knew I could have whatever I really wanted, but in moderation, having it was no longer a big deal or focus in my life. Focus on your health, not your diet.

10. Don't give up when you feel you have slipped. Some people who slip up on a weekend say, "I might as well stay off the bandwagon until Monday." But because you feel you will start depriving yourself on Monday, you overeat. The irony is that most of the time when Monday comes, you tell yourself you'll do it the following Monday, and the cycle continues. Instead of getting caught in the cycle, the very moment you realize your mistake, shake it off, get up, and keep on going. I told you earlier that according to the Bible, those who endure until the end shall be saved. So don't focus on your mistake; focus on your end results.

11. Don't skip meals. Many people think that skipping meals will help them lose weight. But when you skip meals you really set yourself up to overdo it. You are less likely to make healthy choices and may eat more and be willing to grab anything quickly because you're so hungry. It's important to eat at least three meals a day. Eating five or six smaller meals is even better. Eating small, frequent meals actually improves the metabolism.

Being a "diet queen," I used to go all day without eating and thought I was doing great. By the time evening came, I was so hungry I ate whatever I could grab until I was so stuffed I felt intoxicated. Then I went to sleep. The next morning I was too full to eat breakfast and the cycle continued. In the process I actually gained weight. My metabolism was lowered because I had not eaten all day and then I slept on all of those extra calories at night.

12. Read the Bible and pray before you eat. When the devil came to Jesus to tempt Him in the wilderness by urging Him to turn a stone into bread, Jesus' response to him—Matthew 4:4—was *"Man shall not live by bread alone, but by every word that proceeds from the mouth of God."* Although we need physical food to sustain life for the body, we also need spiritual food to sustain life for the soul. I found out that the emptiness or void that I tried to fill with food was actually my spirit needing to be fed the Word of God. The Word is how you find out more about God. Prayer helped me stay in touch with God.

Pray before you eat and ask God, who created your body, to guide you in your eating and give you the strength to not overdo it. When you pray and hear that small still voice tell you you're overdoing it or you've had enough, don't ignore it. Take a deep breath or several if you have to, and then stop. Prayer is very important and it works. But how can you develop a relationship with someone if you never speak to Him? And how can you ever hear His voice for guidance if you never stop to listen?

Although I am giving you tips for trimming the fat, the tips alone didn't help me. One day as I was reading the Bible, I discovered two Scriptures: *"O God, You are my God; early will I seek You; my soul thirsts for You; my flesh longs for You . . ."* (Psalm 63:1); and Psalm 84:2, which reads, *". . . My heart and flesh cry out for the living God."*

In Psalm 63, King David was expressing how intensely lonely he was, and that only God could satisfy his deepest longings. In Psalm

84, the writer expresses his deep desire to be in the presence of God.

I realized that this uncontrollable desire in my flesh, this screaming, burning sensation in my flesh wasn't really about food at all. It was a longing, a desire for God. That's why no matter how much I ate, I was never satisfied; I just got sick. This longing was for the presence of God; it was for the peace of God; it was for the healing of God, which could fulfill and satisfy my soul and my flesh. I once thought that God was interested only in my soul. But when the soul is not satisfied, it will cry out through addictions of the flesh. My problem wasn't about food; it was a "soul thing." That's why it's important to include God in your weight management program.

Look at this Scripture. Proverbs 23:1–3, *"When you sit down to eat with a ruler, consider carefully what is before you; and put a knife to your throat if you are a man given to appetite. Do not desire his delicacies, for they are deceptive food."* Although this Scripture is referring to being careful when eating with someone of power or stature, because he may be trying to bribe you, I see some other symbolism in reference to food. Not only are his delicacies deceptive because of his possible motives; they are also deceptive because of what they can do.

Many of the foods high in calories, sugar, fat, and even sodium are deceptive. They are delicious but can harm you. The Scripture says put a knife to your throat if you have a great appetite. The symbolism I see here in reference to food is that overeating too many of these high-calorie foods is like killing yourself.

Don't consider a weight program that does not promote a healthy lifestyle. The commercials are enticing: "Lose 10 pounds in 10 days, or 5 inches in the same day." If the people promoting these quick fixes cared about your health, they would talk about lifestyle changes and teach you how to take care of yourself.

People constantly call me about these different programs, and many times I want to just burst out and cry. I asked the Lord to please give me the opportunity to tell people the truth. Paul said in Romans 12:1–2, *"I beseech you therefore, brethren, by the mercies of God, that you present your bodies a living sacrifice, holy, and acceptable to God, which is your reasonable service. And do not be conformed to this world, but be transformed by the renewing of your mind, that you may prove what is that good and acceptable and perfect will of God."* I am asking you with all the sincerity in my heart to present your body holy unto God.

Do not run after the quick-fix programs. Do it God's way, which is the only way it can last. The quick-fix programs cause you more harm than good. Many people become seriously ill or their conditions worsen because they took diet pills. Every time you go on one of these quick-fix diets or get your fat "melted away" quickly, your metabolism drops.

Because of the body's protection mechanism that prevents starvation, when you start eating a lot less than what your body needs, your body burns less fat. You do lose weight; however, it is mostly water weight. You also lose lean muscle tissue. Then when you start eating normally again, the pills have lowered your metabolism (the rate at which your body burns fat) and you regain the weight quickly or gain even more weight than you lost. When you try another diet, this cycle repeats itself and you end up in a worse state than you were in before.

Ecclesiastes 10:17 mentions the blessing and importance of eating at regular mealtimes. It reads, *"Blessed are you, O land whose king is of noble birth and whose princes eat at a proper time—for strength and not for drunkenness."*

Think about the long-term effects and your health. Before you go on a fad diet or try a new weight loss program, ask yourself some of these questions: Is it nutritious? Does it include eating a variety of foods to give me sufficient nutrients? Is it a realistic program I can maintain for life? Does it teach me how to live healthier or just focus on quick weight loss? Do they honestly tell me that the recommended healthy weight loss is no more than about one to two pounds per week, or do they promote losing weight quickly? Are the foods for this diet readily available at the grocery store or do I have to buy specific foods? Do I have to rely on a certain type of pill or drink to lose weight rather than focus on health?

Many people fall victim to the vicious cycle of fad dieting and the weight loss trap week after week, month after month, year after year. I was once there myself. I told you earlier I called it a "body trap." I know how it feels to be willing to try almost anything to lose weight. I know how it feels to be so desperate you want to just slice off the fat. I know how it feels to hate your body and not want anyone, not even your own husband, to look at you or touch you.

I was reminded of this recently when I wanted to lose weight again. My body has changed since the first time I lost significant weight. I am no longer in my twenties and I have had surgery on both legs and experience back pain from a car accident. I am forty, and losing weight seems much harder.

Honestly, I was tempted to try one of the fad diets. But I remembered how many people I'd seen lose weight fast then gain it back quickly. Seeing this encouraged me to take my time to do it the right way, not only for long-term results but to feel and look much better. Almost all of the people I've seen on these quick-fix programs do not look vibrant, energetic, and healthy as they are losing weight.

I praise God for the truth. I just cannot stress too much that the only way to lose weight and keep it off is to develop sound eating and exercise habits that you can incorporate into your daily life. Weight lost slowly and gradually is more likely to stay off; weight lost quickly is regained easily. You did not gain the weight overnight, so don't expect to lose it overnight; when you hear of another weight loss program, use the knowledge God is giving you and put that into practice. I strongly encourage all my clients to seek nutrition information. Many health plans now provide nutrition counseling, or you can get a referral for a registered dietitian from your physician. Call the American Dietetic Association (ADA) at their toll-free number, (800) 366-1655, to get health information from their Nutrition Information Line; ask to speak to a registered dietitian (RD) or obtain a referral to one in your area.

Read food labels

It is very important to know what you are eating. Food labels are your best source of information. From the label you'll learn how much fat, sodium, certain nutrients, cholesterol, fiber, and other substances are in foods before you buy them. This will help you make better food selections. Once you read food labels, you will not buy the same.

Many foods have deceptive advertising on the packages or in their names, but the Nutrition Fact Panel on the label tells you the truth. Almost every food in the grocery store will have this information right on its package. The ingredient list is also there to let you know what the food is made of, and in what proportions.

Use these labels also to compare foods. I've done this so much that now it is a habit, and I can do it quickly. We don't have to be ignorant of what we eat anymore; the knowledge is being provided.

You already know that natural foods contain many nutrients that are essential for good health and naturally low in fat. So I will focus on several other items that I feel are important in reducing calories or trimming the fat.

CALORIES

One of the first values listed on a nutrition label is the number of calories contained in the food. I don't count my daily calories; however, I do watch the calories I consume by not eating too many foods high in calories. As we get older our need for calories declines, dropping about 2 percent per decade. Also, when people get older they become less active, which decreases their lean muscle tissue (which helps burn fat). All of this, plus our lowered metabolism, can contribute to extra weight gain. That is why watching your intake of high-calorie foods is very important for weight management.

Reading the food label is a good way to make sure you don't get too many calories. Some people think the way to lose weight is to drastically cut calories. You may be surprised to know that the recommended minimum caloric intake for weight loss is 1,500 to 1,600 calories per day. If you eat a lot less than this, your metabolism may drop too low. You will lose lean muscle tissue and not get enough nutrients for good health.

SERVING SIZE

I think this is one of the most deceptive items on a food label. Most of the serving sizes listed are not the amounts people actually eat. When I teach weight management classes, most people are absolutely amazed when I give them the assignment of bringing in their favorite foods so that we can review the serving sizes listed on the label.

I remember a lady who brought in a small bag of miniature cookies. She thought she was getting very few calories by enjoying the cookies regularly since the label said "150 calories." But she was amazed when I had her take a second look. This time she noticed that the package contained 2.5 servings. Therefore, the amount of calories she was actually consuming by eating this small bag of cookies was 375. And it really wasn't a lot of cookies. I think most people could have eaten two of those small bags. This also meant that the amount of fat and sodium she was consuming was more than twice what she thought.

It is important for you to know that the information listed on the food label applies to only one serving size. If you know you eat more than that, whether the food is nutritious or not, you need to make the correct calculations. So check out the serving size listed on a package to determine what the calories and nutrients really mean to you and your health.

FAT (ESPECIALLY SATURATED FAT)

Although fat can add wonderful flavor and a better texture, and can help you feel more satisfied, you need to watch your intake of fat. A diet high in fat not only contributes to additional pounds but also is not good for your health. One gram of fat has 9 calories, which is more than twice the amount of calories than a gram of protein or carbohydrate. If you read the food label and the food lists 5 grams of fat, the actual amount of calories from the fat is 5 x 9 = 45 calories from fat. If the total calories of the food or serving size is 150 calories, then almost a third of the calories are from fat.

Fat is obvious in some foods such as certain meats, butter, and oil. But there are very many foods in which the fat may not be so obvious: crackers, dairy products, chips, nuts, salad dressing, and many more. The American Heart Association recommends getting no more than 30 percent of your total caloric intake from fats: no more than 10 percent from monounsaturated fats such as nuts, olive oil, or canola oil; about 10 percent from polyunsaturated oil such as corn, soybean, safflower, and sunflower oils; and no more than 10 percent from saturated fats such as animal fats found in meats, whole milk, butter, and coconut and palm oils—two saturated vegetable oils used in many processed foods. Monounsaturated, polyunsaturated, and saturated fat are all listed on the label. The labels have a breakdown of the different fats because diets low in saturated fat (fat that comes from animal products) may decrease the risk of heart disease. The American Heart Association says that eating a diet high in fat (especially saturated fat) and cholesterol is not good for you.

But don't get so hung up on the "fat" on the labels that you do not consider your total calorie intake. For instance, many foods have "low fat" listed on their packages, but they are high in sugar and calories. And extra calories, whether from fat or sugar, put extra fat on the body.

CHOLESTEROL

Although cholesterol is not fat, it is a fatlike substance. Fat and cholesterol are sometimes used together or often thought of as being the same substance because they normally appear together in foods of animal origin. Also, both fat and cholesterol are often considered "bad," but both are also important in the body.

Cholesterol is part of every cell in the body and helps the body digest fat. Cholesterol in the skin turns to vitamin D, an essential nutrient, when exposed to sunlight. There are two types of cholesterol. Blood or serum cholesterol is found in our blood. Dietary cholesterol is found in the food we eat. The body makes its own cholesterol in the liver, but also the animal products we eat such as meat, eggs, poultry, fish, and dairy products contain cholesterol. Eating foods high in dietary cholesterol can raise the blood cholesterol levels in some people. High blood cholesterol is a risk factor for heart disease and related illnesses. To watch your intake of cholesterol, eat no more than four egg yolks per week, eat leaner meat, poultry, and fish, and eat low-fat dairy products. Organ meats such as liver are high in cholesterol, so watch your consumption of organ meats. There is no Recommended Dietary Allowance (RDA) for cholesterol; however, the guideline for healthy adults is 300 milligrams or less per day.

SODIUM

The sodium content of some of the foods you purchase or eat will surprise you. Make it a habit to look at the sodium content on food labels. I avoid buying many foods, especially many prepared foods, because they are so high in sodium. Again, it is important to look at the serving size and estimate the amount you will eat to get an accurate calculation of your sodium intake. Remember: 500 milligrams of sodium is the estimated minimum amount to keep the body operating smoothly, and 2,400 milligrams or less of sodium per day has been advised for healthy adults.

Be sure to read the label to find out the ingredients in what you are eating. Ingredients are listed in order, with the first being the ingredient present in the greatest amount and the last being present in the least amount. Look for foods that list more wholesome natural products first. Also, beware of foods listing a lot of artificial ingredients. If you can't recognize an ingredient or pronounce it, ask yourself how natural it can be.

Listen to your body

Have you ever eaten until you were so full you had to unbutton your pants or felt like you had to take a nap? Your body was trying to tell you something.

Long before people counted calories and read food labels, there was a simple way to determine whether you needed to eat or had eaten too much. It was to listen to your body. When God created the human body He didn't make any mistakes. He created the body with internal signals. Can you imagine how it would be if we never got the signal we were hungry—or satisfied? We would die of starvation or eat ourselves to death.

One of the reasons I was able to stop counting calories is that I learned to listen to my body. I used to eat until I felt as if I had taken a sedative or was so tired and sluggish that I had to lie down and take a nap. When I tried diet programs, I felt light-headed, irritable, and weak, and at other times I had stomach cramps. My body was talking to me. In one case it told me I was overeating and had gotten too many calories, and in the other instance it told me I wasn't eating enough.

Listening to your body will help you avoid overeating or eating too many high-calorie foods. Here are more tips:

EAT WHEN YOU'RE HUNGRY

Your stomach may feel empty or even grumble. Many people eat for reasons other than hunger—because the food is there, out of habit, because they think it's time to eat since others are eating, or for emotional or spiritual reasons, as I mentioned before.

Do you normally eat because your body told you to, or do you eat out of habit? When was the last time your stomach grumbled? Let your body guide you.

DON'T KEEP EATING UNTIL YOU'RE OVERFULL

This is a big problem for most of us who struggle to lose weight. Instead of eating until we are satisfied, we tend to eat until we are full. Then we get sluggish because we overate. This habit starts at a very young age. We feed babies until they are nice and full, so they can go to sleep. Some people even give their babies cereal at a very young age so that they will get full and sleep longer through the night. Some of us were told as children to eat all of the food on our plates. We have taken this message into our adult lives: cleaning our plates, eating until we have to loosen our pants, and then going back for seconds and thirds. Some people even wear pants with elastic in the waist when they go to all-you-can-eat restaurants, determined to eat all they can and get their money's worth. Still, we wonder why we have a midsection bulge.

EAT SLOWLY

Eating too fast is a sure way of overeating. It takes about twenty minutes for the brain to get the message that you have eaten. If you eat faster than that, you are more likely to overeat. You will continue to feel hungry because your body hasn't gotten the message that you have eaten.

So slow down and chew thoroughly. Cut your food into small pieces and drink water between bites if you have to.

ENJOY YOUR FOOD

Listen to your taste buds. I had to learn how to enjoy my food so I wouldn't overeat. Eating should be a very important time of the day. Food is for life, yet we often take it for granted. I stopped talking on the phone, watching television, and working during lunch so I could enjoy the taste of my foods.

Many people tell me they overeat late at night because that is the only time they get to enjoy the taste of food. Don't rush your breakfast, and don't inhale your lunch. Take the time to sit down, relax, and enjoy your food, even if it means extra time. Many people work through lunch and have to pay the price later. They go home and overeat, then go to bed.

LEARN HOW FOOD AFFECTS YOU

I felt better and lighter when I stopped eating so many high-calorie and fattening foods. Foods high in fat can be tasty and satisfying but they also make you feel less energetic. I woke up more easily when I didn't eat a lot of fattening foods. I paid attention and discovered how specific foods affected me.

There is a good Scripture that refers to overeating. Proverbs 23:20–21: *"Do not mix with wine bibbers, or with gluttonous eaters of meat; for the drunkard and the glutton will come to poverty, and drowsiness will clothe a man with rags."*

In this passage of the Bible, gluttony and drunkenness are used in the same regard as having the same effect. I can truly relate to this passage. I did not get drunk off of liquor often, but overindulging in food created a similar state for me.

Many Christians feel their lives are in order because they no longer participate in those activities "of the world" that they consider wrong such as getting drunk, using drugs, or having sex. But for many it is as though food has taken the place of those other desires. Churches frequently have activities in which food is served or sold. And I haven't seen a fruit or salad bar there yet. In the church, it seems as though food has become the center of joy, or an outlet for many people. I even had someone who was extremely overweight tell me that she doesn't have sex, so she was going to enjoy herself by indulging in food.

Perhaps eating seems so innocent because we need food for life; therefore, it is easy for people to indulge themselves without feeling as though they are harming their bodies. But food can have a detrimental effect on your health, on your total well-being, and on God being able to use you to your full potential. Prepare your holy temple correctly.

The bottom line is that it is up to you. You have a choice to make. I have overextended myself many times trying to help others. I had to learn that people must want health for themselves. I couldn't be God and Savior for anyone. I couldn't even help myself. It took the power of God to help me. I made a decision to live a healthy life, and I was willing to make the necessary changes to achieve that goal.

There is a story in Luke 14:24–34 regarding making a choice. At this point, Jesus' popularity was widespread, and he was like a celebrity. Literally thousands of people followed Him to hear Him speak and see Him perform His many miracles. But not all of these people were true disciples of Christ.

On this particular occasion Jesus confronted the crowd. He explained to them that it may pay to serve Christ, but it also comes with a cost. He explained that certain conditions have to be met in order to be a disciple of Christ. In verses 28–33 he uses parables about counting the cost of discipleship. He uses these illustrations to show that every goal or accomplishment requires careful consideration. So instead of just following Christ, you need to first think about whether or not you are willing to do what it takes to follow Christ. This may mean giving up your own desires and giving up every corner of your life or "you cannot be Christ's disciple" (verse 33). Many people came to hear his teaching, but when Jesus made it clear that certain directives must be followed in order to be a disciple, some people withdrew from following him.

What does this story have to do with weight management? Many people want to lose weight and look and feel better, but everyone seems to be looking for a quick-fix method, as they did with Jesus. Everyone wanted to be healed and reap the benefits of His kingdom, but many didn't want to do what it takes to truly live for Christ. If you truly want to lose weight, keep it off, and look and feel better, you have to make a choice that you are willing to do it the right way. Doing it God's way includes developing healthier eating habits, taking the time to care for your body, and going to God in prayer and asking for His guidance.

Although discipleship may come with a cost, the benefits are far greater. To have joy, peace, hope, and eternal life with God forever is far greater than any sacrifice that could be made. Likewise, to have a more fulfilling, energetic, vibrant life and to live life to the fullness of your purpose by committing to healthier living is far greater than any sacrifice you could make. What will it really cost you to care for the temple of God? Your reward will be so much greater.

Continue to read this book, then go back to each week and try to incorporate the necessary changes into your life. Don't forget the story of Joshua, the children of Israel, and the Promised Land. Joshua and the Israelites conquered the land in sections until they had conquered it all. Don't get stuck on one week you find particularly challenging. Move on and improve and come back to that week if you have to.

Remember, those who are the most successful are those who start out slowly, making gradual changes and not giving up. Allow the Lord to order your steps so that you can learn how to be "fit for God."

Prayer

Say this prayer with me.

Dear God,
I am making the decision right now to live a healthy life. I want
to be free from the bondage of food so I can feel better and live a
life full of vitality, hope, peace, and joy. Fill me with your love;
fill me with your peace and your joy so the longing in my soul and

flesh can be satisfied. Calm my spirit and ease my mind so the craving in my body will be put to rest. Surround me in your presence and heal my hurts and pains so food will no longer be my comfort and friend. I need your help, I need your guidance, and I need your comfort. In Jesus' name I pray. Amen

Study Scriptures

PROVERBS 23:1–3

When you sit down to eat with a ruler, consider carefully what is before you; and put a knife to your throat if you are a man given to appetite. Do not desire his delicacies, for they are deceptive food.

MATTHEW 5:6

Blessed are those who hunger and thirst for righteousness, for they shall be filled.

ACTIVITIES

1. From your food journal, make a list of the high-fat, high-sugar, or high-sodium foods you eat, using the information from this week's lesson.

2. What are some of the changes you could make based on the list of tips given this week?

3. Start off making one realistic change at a time. For example, replace a high-fat food with a healthier alternative (examples: bake chicken instead of fry, use 1 percent milk instead of whole milk, have a bagel for breakfast instead of a donut, or fruit with lunch instead of chips).

EXERCISE

Many people complain about boredom while exercising. So this week, change your workout routine, your scenery—or both. For instance, instead of using dumbbells to strengthen your muscles, use an exercise band or tube or find something in your home to use. You can use soup cans, books, or even a towel to strengthen muscles, and you can do toe raises on the stairs to develop your calf muscles. Instead of walking around a track or on the treadmill, walk around the neighborhood. Instead of going to the gym, try the jogging and biking trails at a park.

When was the last time you enjoyed the sights in your city? Park the car or ride the bus or subway and go sightseeing. Ask friends, your husband, the kids, or your coworkers for suggestions of other enjoyable activities or places to go to break your old routine and add excitement to your exercise life. How about skating, swimming, softball, volleyball, canoeing, or horseback riding? Have fun learning a new activity or walking where you have never walked before.

Get rid of the excuses that may stop you from being "fit for God"

1. MARRIAGE

Many people get married and all of a sudden feel so comfortable they no longer take care of their health. Whatever you did to get your spouse, you shouldn't stop once you're married. God didn't create marriage so that we could develop poor health habits. He created it so that man and woman could be a blessing to one another and find favor from the Lord. Encourage (don't nag) your spouse to live a healthier life. **Proverbs 18:22** *He who finds a wife finds a good thing, and obtains favor from the Lord.*

2. LACK OF EXERCISE

Health experts concur that one of the main reasons people struggle with obesity and certain preventable illnesses is the lack of activity. Although you should exercise because it produces wonderful benefits for the body, your primary focus should be exercising your spirit mainly through obedience to God. So get up and move your body and soul! **I Timothy 4:8** *For bodily exercise profits a little, but godliness is profitable for all things, having the promise of the life that now is and of that which is to come.*

3. LACK OF JOY

If you don't seem to have any joy in your life, check out the company you're keeping and how you're spending your time. If you spend adequate time with God, you will be overwhelmed with joy because you are in the presence of the lover of your soul. **Psalm 16:11** *You will show me the path of life; in Your presence is the fullness of joy; at your right hand are pleasures forevermore.*

4. "I DO WELL DURING THE DAY AND THEN I GET REALLY HUNGRY AND OVERDO IT AT NIGHT"

Most of us who have struggled with losing weight probably understand this. You think that the best way to lose weight is to *not* eat. So you don't eat breakfast, try to eat very little or nothing at all for lunch, and then in the evening—once you put the first bite of food in your mouth—you are absolutely out of control. You overindulge until you are stuffed. Then you tell yourself you are not going to lose control the next day, but you repeat the vicious cycle anyway. The problem is, you have to eat if you want to lose weight, and you have to eat if you want to maintain control. Experts recommend eating at least four to six small meals a day to keep your metabolism active and prevent hunger pangs and uncontrollable urges. You need to make sure you eat at least three meals throughout the day, with breakfast or lunch being the heavier meals. You can also snack in between, with light snacks or fruit counting as the additional meals. In order to have control at night, you have to take control and eat during the day. **Matthew 6:11** *Give us this day our daily bread.*

5. "I OVEREAT DURING HOLIDAYS, SOCIAL EVENTS, OR AT OFFICE PARTIES"

Food has long been part of many gatherings, festive celebrations, and family events for cultures all over the world. Many people gain at least five to seven pounds during the holidays. One way to avoid overeating at a social event is to not go to the event hungry. Eat a light meal before you go. At the event, first fill up on the healthier foods like salads and vegetables, and drink plenty of water with your meal. Get smaller plates and smaller serving sizes. You can always take leftovers home from a restaurant. At the office, suggest bagels instead of donuts, and fruit and vegetable trays instead of snack trays. On the day you know you are going to eat all of your favorite foods, eat a light breakfast and lunch. You don't have to eat everything at one sitting either; eat a series of small meals. Use common sense. God made us to have fellowship with one another, and "breaking bread" together is a great way to enjoy family and friends. **I John 1:7** *But if we walk in the light as He is in the light, we have fellowship with one another, and the blood of Jesus Christ His Son cleanses us from all sin.*

6. "I DON'T WANT TO GIVE UP MY FAVORITE FOODS"

I would have been delivered from overeating a long time ago if I had known the truth: Giving up all of your favorites is a sure way to set yourself up for bingeing. What I have discovered is that the problem isn't necessarily the types of food we eat, but *how much* of these foods we eat. And when you do eat these foods, don't quickly gulp them down. Take your time and savor every bite so that you will be less likely to get seconds. As I said earlier in this chapter, pick a particular day of the week that will be your day to enjoy some of your favorite foods. If you really want something, don't keep eating substitutes only to be dissatisfied and find yourself eating what you wanted anyway. **I Corinthians 9:25** *And everyone who competes for the prize is temperate in all things. Now they do it to obtain a perishable crown, but we for an imperishable crown.*

Week Six
Don't Try to Do It Alone

So God Created Man in His Own Image; in the Image of
God He Created Him; Male and Female He Created Them.
—Genesis 1:27

O n the sixth day the earth is the right distance from the sun;
there is day and night, time, seasons, and years. The water
is ready for man to drink, oxygen is in the air for him to
breathe, the vegetation is ready for him to eat, and the animals are
under his authority. The earth is now ready to be inhabited by God's
ultimate creation. When God made all of these things before He
created humans, He said *"Let there be,"* and whatever He spoke
came into existence. However, when it was time for His ultimate
creation, God did something different. This creation wasn't like anything else He had previously made.

It was almost as if God were preparing a stage with all the right
props and the proper lighting for the star of a show. When it was time
for the star, a human, to come forward, everything was done completely differently. This was the first and only creation that God
made in His image, and the only time in Scripture He says *"Let Us
make . . ."* Unlike what some scientists would have you believe, the
universe is not the major story in creation. Man is the star of this
show. God clearly gives that implication by not focusing on how He
created the universe, and by doing what He had *not* done previously.

God is not physical, but spiritual, so man was not made in God's physical image. And although God is infinite and man is finite, man was made to possess the characteristics or attributes of God. He was given intellect, the ability to reason, the ability to make decisions, and to have morals and values, unlike the animals. He was made to think and have feelings. He was also made to have the creative ability of God, and other attributes to reflect the image of God such as wisdom, knowledge, love, kindness, and forgiveness. Mankind is very special to God. Every human being should know that he or she is special just because God thought so much of him to make him in His very own image.

Our self-worth should not depend on our material possessions— our education, how much money we make, our occupations, where we live, what type of car we drive, and so on, but on the fact that we are special to the Almighty God, the Eternal Creator of heaven and earth.

Despite what evolutionists believe, man did not evolve. We did not originate from an amoeba, fish, or ape. To accept that theory is like me telling you that I got pregnant by swallowing a watermelon seed. It is ludicrous. Because man's intellectual ability cannot match or come close to the sovereignty and omnipotence of God, he has to guess what he thinks happened. But the Bible, which is the inspired Word of God, the word that God breathed into men to record, the word that is historically accurate, clearly states that man was created by God, not over a period of time. Instead, *"The Lord God formed man from the dust of the ground, and breathed into his nostrils the breath of life; and man became a living being"* (Genesis 2:7).

When God made the first man, Adam, the Bible says that God said, *"It is not good that man should be alone; I will make him a helper comparable to him."* So God put Adam into a deep sleep and took one of his ribs and closed up the flesh. From the rib He took from man, God made a woman (Genesis 2:18–25).

Imagine Adam seeing for the first time the amazing array of creatures, the colorful exotic birds and huge fruit trees, fresh springs of water, and multitude of flowers. He had to notice that there was more than one of everything—a Mr. and Mrs. Elephant, a Mr. and Mrs. Giraffe, a Mr. and Mrs. Duck, that even ants had families, and so on. As Adam was naming all the animals, he had to realize that there was no one else like him, and he was alone. Whether he thought about it or not, I guess, can be debated. But God clearly stated that it wasn't good for Adam to be alone. God's work of creation was not complete without woman.

The New King James Version of the Bible says God made man a "helper," and the King James Version (Genesis 2:18) says "help meet." Both versions imply that Adam needed some help and was not to take care of God's creation alone. And God did not take the bone from which he made woman from one of Adam's feet, which could symbolically represent woman being under his feet or him being able to walk all over her. He did not take the bone from one of his hands, which some could interpret as giving him a right to hit her; nor did He take it from his head, in which case she would be over him. But God—in his creative wisdom—took her right from the side of man to walk beside him and complement him in a mutual, loving union.

You may be wondering what God creating man and woman has to do with weight management. When God created the universe He did not do it alone. When God created Adam, He did not leave him alone, and don't you try to do it alone, either. Adam could talk directly to God, yet he still needed help. You, too, are going to need help, encouragement, and support from others.

One day the Lord placed on my heart to call Betty, a participant in one of my previous Fit for God weight management workshops. She said it was amazing that I called since she was feeling bad about overeating and not sticking to her exercise program. When Betty had shared her testimony on my local cable program *Eternally Fit,* I had asked her what really helped her maintain a healthy living. She told me that knowing she had the help of God and having an exercise partner were the things that kept her going. So on the day I called, I asked her if she had been praying or listening to the voice of God, and if she was keeping in touch with her partner.

She answered "no" to each question. She had gotten a promotion and was so caught up in the new job that she was slack in her fitness program. She was making the extra money she wanted, but her health was paying for it. I prayed with her and strongly encouraged her to always make the time to commune with God and to also get in touch with her fitness partner again.

She called me back weeks later and said she was back on track.

Here are three suggestions so that you won't have to go through your Fit for God program alone:

1. PRAY AND ASK GOD TO LEAD YOU TO A FITNESS PARTNER.

Just think about it. Though Adam could speak to God, God still felt it was best for Adam to have somebody like him by his side. Betty, the client I mentioned earlier, stated that having a partner helped tremendously to keep her on track and committed to her program. Some studies even suggest that married people live longer than single people, and it is often recommended that a person get a pet rather than live completely alone. As great and awesome as God is, He is not alone and was not alone in the very beginning of creation when He said, *"Let Us make man . . ."*

I believe creation worked something like this: God was the architect, Jesus was the supplier, and the Holy Spirit did the actual construction, or was the builder. They worked in unity to accomplish this magnificent task.

Being a loner was one of my biggest problems and made my struggle to lose weight more difficult. People often have prayer partners for their souls, but because we have a tripartite nature, we still need to take care of the body. Frequently, as was the case with my-self, neglect of the temple is caused by a spiritual issue. So in actu-ality, your prayer partner could also be your fitness partner.

My prayer partner and I could not work out together as much as I would have liked, because we both had families and very busy schedules. But she was still a fitness partner in many instances. When I got the urge to overeat or neglect my health, I called her and she encouraged me until the desire to overindulge subsided. Like-wise, I often encouraged her to eat right and exercise. When one of us was down or didn't feel like taking care of her health, the other provided the inspiration. When we did exercise together, it was a very positive experience.

Having this relationship was truly a blessing for me because in the past I was so ashamed of my overeating that I tried to handle the problem by myself. But I constantly failed until I accepted the fact that I needed to be honest with myself and with others: I needed help. Having a relationship with others, without the shame, was the beginning step toward my success.

The Bible has a lot to say about relationships. The Ten Com-mandments were even about relationships. The first set of com-mandments involves a relationship with God, the next involves a relationship with the family, and the last set involves relationships with others.

In Jesus' teachings He also addresses the importance of relation-ships with others. When a lawyer asked Him what was the greatest commandment, He replied, *"You shall love the Lord with all your heart . . . and you shall love your neighbor as yourself"* (Matthew 22:37–40).

In the book of Philippians, Chapter 2, the apostle Paul speaks of the importance of people coming together in unity, and how we should not only be concerned for our own interests but also look out for the interest of others. And in Galatians 6:2, Paul states that we ought to bear one another's burdens. So get rid of your pride and get a partner.

As far as finding a fitness "buddy," you don't want to grab just anyone. Pray and ask God to lead you to the right person. Does your partner have to be highly motivated, knowledgeable in health and fitness, and in great athletic condition? Do you just need to hire a personal trainer?

The answer to those questions is "no." Having a personal trainer is great to get you started and to get you on a program designed specifically for you, but not everyone can afford a trainer. And while we personal trainers motivate and educate, our primary objective is for clients to be able to successfully live healthy without the trainer. Even if you have a trainer, a partner is still great for those times when you need encouragement and the trainer is not around.

When you choose a partner, it is important to find one who has goals similar to yours: to live healthier by eating right, to exercise, and to take care of the whole person—spirit, soul, and body. You do not want a partner who is a hindrance to your progress. If your partner is always negative or wants to eat out too often, you may want to initially encourage this person to live healthier. But if there is no change over a period of time, find another partner.

God made Eve a helper to Adam. If Adam needed help, Eve was right there by his side. So you also need someone by your side, not hanging on to your coattails or dragging you down.

Don't misconstrue what I mean. You and your partner do not have to be at the same fitness level. You may be in better physical condition than your partner, or your partner may have a healthier diet than you do. It doesn't matter who is doing better or how. You simply want someone who is striving to go in the right direction.

The Bible says, *"How can two walk together unless they agree?"* (Amos 3:3). So you need to at least agree on the goal.

Another benefit of getting a partner is having someone to be accountable to. Knowing that you made an appointment to work out with someone can help you stay on course. Having a partner can also push you to work harder. Even when I was tired and ready to stop, I pushed myself to continue when my partner was present. Ultimately, having a partner can help you reach your goal faster.

One of the reasons why I suggest praying and asking God to direct you to the right partner is because you may want to share your eating habits and some of your notes from your journal with your partner. It is not absolutely necessary that you share all of your notes, but you do want to establish some type of trust and accountability.

James 5:16 reads, *"Confess your trespasses to one another, and pray for one another, that you may be healed. The effective fervent prayer of a righteous man avails much."*

Although we can go directly to God in prayer, sharing our struggles with a partner provides support that will also help us overcome challenges. I shared some of my notes with my partner, and together we came up with solutions as we searched through Scriptures. We also shared what we ate, and this is where the accountability part really affected me the most. There were times when I wanted to overeat, but because I knew I had to share with my partner, I didn't eat everything I wanted. To my surprise, one day when my partner and I were talking, she told me she didn't eat everything she wanted to either because she knew she had to share that information with me. Finally, she said she no longer had the desire to eat the amount of chocolate candy she normally ate each day. So accountability forced us to eat healthier and avoid overindulging until healthy eating became a habit.

Adam and Eve were accountable to God when they were in the Garden of Eden. Although you may have your partner for accountability, remember that ultimately you too are accountable to God for all of your actions, including neglect of His temple. So you might as well be honest with yourself; there is no way to keep a secret from

God. If you need help, ask God to help you stick to your program and lead you to the right partner.

2. SHARE YOUR HEALTHIER LIVING GOALS WITH YOUR FAMILY AND FRIENDS

God made us to be gregarious. You cannot avoid socializing or being with your family, friends, and loved ones. Let them know what you are doing and why it's important to you. Wanting to be healthy or to lose weight is nothing to be ashamed of and should be something we want to share, especially with those closest to us. I know many people who say they don't want to share with anyone, that they only want people to see their results.

But for whom are you really doing it? If you are doing it for you, you don't need to show anybody anything. And by letting them know, you may receive additional support.

Claire is a client I shared this with because she was concerned about keeping her weight program a secret until she shed enough pounds for people to notice. Consequently, she was often tempted to overeat because her children dropped by with her favorite half gallon of ice cream, her godmother made her favorite cake, and one of the church mothers made her apple pies. She didn't refuse the foods because at the time she was not strong enough to say no or to eat them in moderation.

I encouraged her to let those around her know that she really wanted to live healthier. I also told her that if they wanted to bring her snacks—because she worked long hours on her job—she should suggest they bring fresh fruit or salad.

She finally shared her goals with others. Her children were happy for her because she was substantially overweight, and they wanted their mother happy and healthy. It even changed her husband's behavior because he knew his wife needed to be healthier, and he wanted to help. He was a naturally slim person and worked out regularly, but he loved snacks as well. When she told him what she was trying to do, he stopped bringing snacks home. When I asked him if he was giving up his favorite snacks entirely, he laughed and said, "No, I just eat them at work before I come home."

Claire also shared her health goals with the church members, and many of them joined her in trying to live healthier by changing their diets and exercising more. When she shared her challenge with people on her job, instead of always buying donuts they started buying bagels and fresh fruits.

Claire created awareness in her home, on her job, and at church that eating the right foods and exercising is important. She was a very powerful witness to many people because they actually saw the results of her weight program.

Many times we think it is a treat to give kids junk food, to make goodies for people, or to indulge in certain foods ourselves. We need to find other ways to show our appreciation and treat ourselves. Yes, food is for life and to be enjoyed, but it shouldn't be the only way to create something positive for you or others. You can give kids fruit, fruit pops, or fruit shakes; you can also take them to the park, go walking with them, or rent a video. Most of the time what they really want anyway is attention and love. Giving kids a lollipop for bringing in their homework or baking someone a cake or pie is a nice and thoughtful gesture, but in the long run, is it really contributing to their well-being? You can treat others with a card, a fruit basket, or just some words of encouragement or a nice warm smile. Use your creativity and discover other treats of life.

Obesity is considered an epidemic in our society. We need to stop focusing on our personal goals and issues and start thinking collectively and corporately. Don't try to get fit alone, and don't allow others to do it all alone. God never intended for us to live that way. Remember: The whole Bible is about relationships. When Paul addressed the church in the book of Ephesians, he was speaking of relationships. In Ephesians 4:16 he describes the church as consisting of a body of individual parts (people) who all do their share for the growth of the church.

In Ephesians, Chapters 5 and 6, Paul addresses relationships, including those within the family, which is the role model for the church of God. In I Corinthians, Chapter 12, beginning at verse 12, Paul compares the church to the human body. The church consists of many members of one body with each part being important and having a specific function for the body as a whole. Just as the eyes are for seeing, the ears for hearing, the legs for walking, and the other members have their specific roles, people were created to work together for the common good of all mankind. Each of us has specific gifts and talents that can benefit or help others. When you try to do it alone, not only do you miss your blessing but you also miss out on being a blessing to someone else.

One of the greatest joys I have experienced in my life is when I have been able to make a positive difference in someone else's life. If I'm not helping someone, I don't feel the true fullness of what I think life should be.

There is really no excuse for any human being to be alone. Do you want a friend? The Bible says that a person who has friends must himself be friendly (Proverbs 18:24). Some people walk around looking so mean or depressed that no one wants to know them. Even some Christians walk around looking like they suck on lemons all day. Why would anyone want to befriend them?

Pray and ask God to reveal a true friend to you or send one to you. If you don't have a friendly disposition, pray and ask God to make you a friendlier and more pleasant person who will attract true friends. God doesn't want you alienated from anyone. Reach out and tell others you need their support, make yourself friendly, and experience the joy of not having to do it all by yourself.

Staying alone and trying to work everything out on my own almost caused me to lose my mind and my health. Not only did I one day find myself traveling down a long, dark path of despair and depression, but I also struggled with having no control over my eating habits year after year. Once I began talking to others and allowed them to show me support, I was released from my shame, anxiety, and depression. The Bible says that pride comes before a fall or destruction (Proverbs 16:18), and my pride almost caused me my mental and physical health.

When God sent Moses to tell Pharaoh to let His people go from bondage in the land of Egypt, Moses didn't go alone. Aaron, his brother, went with him. When the Messiah, Jesus Christ the Son of the Living God, started His public ministry, He didn't do it alone. He chose twelve disciples and had an inner circle of Peter, James, and John, with whom He spent a lot of time. When He sent His disciples out to travel from town to town spreading the gospel, He sent them out in groups of twos.

The Bible stresses the strength we have in numbers. For instance, the Word of God says when two or three gather together in God's name, He is right there in the midst. So when you get together with others, God's presence and power to accomplish whatever you need shows up right there.

Also take a look at God's multiplication or addition. The Bible says that one can put a thousand to flight but two can put ten thousand to flight. It would seem logical that if one can put one thousand to flight, then two can put two thousand to flight. But God is clearly showing that when we get together we can do much more than if we try alone.

This reminds me of working out. For instance, when I do single-arm dumbbell curls, I may use a 15-pound dumbbell on each arm. But when I use the curl bar, in which both arms are lifting the weight simultaneously, I use at least 40 pounds. The logical weight to use would seem to be 30 pounds, but when I use both arms I can do more than twice the amount of one arm. This is true when I lift weights with my legs as well. God works this way with us. Many great things can happen when we get together, for He designed us to be with one another and help each other.

In the Bible we also find examples of the detrimental effect being alone can have on a human being: Elijah, whose story is in I Kings and II Kings, is the prophet who didn't die. He was taken away by a chariot of fire up to heaven in a whirlwind. He was a great man of God, and God used him to perform a number of miracles. The most frequently taught miracle is that of the widow's handful of flour and little bit of oil in a jar, which were multiplied during a drought. The widow and her son had only enough flour and oil to bake one more small cake. They were going to eat it, then lie down and die of starvation. But because she obeyed the word of Elijah, given to him by God, God multiplied her little bit and she had an unending supply of food throughout the drought.

Other miracles of Elijah include being fed by ravens, raising the widow's son from the dead, calling fire down from heaven to consume the altar of the false god and those who opposed him, and parting the Red Sea. Elijah spoke a word and the heavens shut up and there was a drought throughout the land. Then he spoke again and the rain returned.

Elijah was mightily used by God and saw the miraculous power of God being worked through him. Yet Elijah often had to stand alone in his ministry and sometimes face hundreds by himself. This great man of faith couldn't fathom loneliness and despair; he became depressed and wanted to die when he thought he was alone. Elijah actually prayed to God to let him die. He thought all the other prophets had been killed and he was the only one left. But an angel of God told him to get up, eat, and drink something to get some strength. Elijah then prayed to God, and the Lord assured him there were thousands like him left who didn't worship the false gods. God in His faithfulness answered Elijah's prayer, directed him to the other prophets, and led him to his traveling companion and successor, Elisha.

There will be times when you feel alone in your struggle, but don't give up. Don't throw in the towel. Many people just like you have gone through some of the very same things you have.

I'm telling you right now, you don't have to be prepared to lie down and die, or give up. This applies to whatever you are going through. As long as there is life, there is always hope. With the Almighty God on your side, you cannot fail. The only person who can stop you is you. The only person who can keep you down is you. The widow and her son believed in their hearts that there was no hope for them. But when she listened to the prophet of God and tried what he said, the miraculous happened. When Elijah wanted to give up and die, he prayed to God, and God led him to others like himself. Remember, with God all things are possible.

3. Feel the Spirit; know that God is with you

What if God hasn't led you to those true friends or your fitness partner yet? What if you don't have many friends or family members you can really share with, or if no one is available or around? Do you just accept the fact that you are all alone?

Feel the Spirit. Know that God is with you.

In the Book of Joshua, Chapter 1, Moses is dead and Joshua, his assistant, has succeeded him. After the people mourned Moses, God told Joshua it was time for them to get up and go and conquer the land. Joshua was traveling with an entire nation of people, yet God told him twice in Chapter 1 that He was with him. Joshua 1:5 reads, ". . . *I will not leave you nor forsake you,*" and Joshua 1:9 reads, ". . . *Be strong and of good courage; do not be afraid, nor be dismayed, for the Lord your God is with you wherever you go.*"

At first I used to wonder why God told Joshua three times in one chapter to be strong and courageous. Then I realized God knew that this would seem like a difficult task. He didn't want Joshua to become discouraged, which is a normal human emotion when presented with great challenges. Because God knew this, He assured Joshua repeatedly that he would never be alone, that He would always be with him to direct him and help fight his battles.

Just as God was with Joshua and the children of Israel, you need to also know beyond a shadow of a doubt that God is with you. God doesn't change, so today He is still able to help His children overcome any and all battles. But He can't help you if you don't let him. One thing I love about God is that He doesn't force us to do anything. He gave us a free will. I believe that's one of the reasons why God allows evil to exist. I have spoken to people who often wonder why such a good God allows evil to exist. I personally believe one of the reasons is that its existence gives His creation a free choice. We have the choice to listen to God and follow His directives or do things in a way we think is right, which often can lead to despair, failure, and regret. God gave Joshua specific instructions for conquering the land; however, it was up to Joshua to follow God's instructions.

If you are to overcome the battle of the bulge, you have to know that God is with you, He will never leave you, and He will guide you to victory if you let Him.

Jim was a personal client who struggled with losing weight most of his life. When he first came to me, his diet was absolutely horrendous. He actually referred to himself as "the fast-food king" because most of his meals were from fast-food restaurants. In addition, he drank sodas all day, didn't drink water, snacked constantly, and didn't eat any fruits and vegetables. Of course, he was overweight and had high blood pressure. He specifically wanted help because he had tried other programs but just couldn't stay motivated to lose weight and stick to a fitness regimen.

As I talked to him more, it was obvious that food was Jim's comfort and friend and that it validated his existence as a human being.

He was a very lonely man, an only child raised by a single mother, who was now deceased. He had barely had a relationship with his father, who had also died. He was divorced and didn't have many friends. Working out and exercising regularly did wonders for Jim physically, but he still struggled with his food addiction.

Jim had attended Christian school when he was younger, believed in God, and went to church occasionally. He didn't understand or have a concept of God being available to help His children overcome any type of problem or struggle in life. He was a very proud man, college educated and quite successful in his career, so he relied on himself and no one else. He had survived the pain and disappointments in his life, yet he still couldn't control his eating.

It wasn't hard for me to realize that food was not Jim's problem. Although I gave him a workout regimen and some healthy tips for eating right, I also began to minister God's Word to him. Jim rededicated his life to Christ, but still often felt empty inside and all alone. I expressed to him many times that he was not alone, that God was with him. I told him that whatever he was searching for could be found only through God. But because he couldn't see a physical being or hear a loud voice, he had a difficult time grasping the concept that God was truly with him and was able to guide him in every area of his life, including his eating habits.

I suggested that Jim do something I used to do when I felt the onset of one of my anxiety attacks and the mad, uncontrollable craving to eat. I would stop doing whatever I was about to do, whether it was grab a sandwich or a bag of chips, cookies, or ice cream. I would pause, and take at least three long, deep breaths. I would inhale and exhale slowly. This would clear my mind and relax me long enough to stop me from overindulging. It also gave me time to pray and listen to God direct me in my eating habits before I found myself in another binge cycle.

When I initially told Jim to do this, he thought it was a little strange. But with absolutely nothing to lose, he tried it and found that it helped him in a number of ways. First, he said, it made him focus on his weight loss and health goals, which helped him stop the uncontrollable eating. Second, it gave him time to realize he wasn't alone, that God was with him and available to guide him.

I like to say, "As long as there is life there is hope." So I told him that taking the deep breaths were symbolic of that life. And anytime you have life, you have the opportunity to overcome any problem. Just knowing that you have that life should let you know undoubtedly that God is with you because it is God who is the giver of that life.

Jim grew into this truth. Whenever he felt the urge to overindulge in the wrong foods, he took deep breaths, which allowed him to "feel the Spirit" and know that God is always with him.

Genesis 2:7 says, *"And the Lord God formed man of the dust of the ground, and breathed into his nostrils the breath of life; and man became a living being."*

God formed man from the dust of the ground, but man still did not have life. His heart wasn't pumping, his blood wasn't circulating, and his brain was not sending electrical impulses or messages anywhere. But when God breathed His breath of life into man's nostrils, then man became a living being. The word used in the Old Testament for breath or spirit is *ruach,* which has as its basic meaning "something that is unseen, yet powerful and full of life-giving qualities." It can be interpreted as the "life-force" or the "breath of God."

Not only did God breathe into Adam's nostrils so that he might live, but when we wake up each morning it's because God has kept His breath of life flowing throughout our respiratory systems. When He takes it back or removes it, then life as we know it ceases. This breath belongs to God, it comes from God, and is part of God. Therefore, every human being who is alive on the face of the earth has a piece of our Creator. If you are alive, God is aware of your existence, knows who you are, and is available to help you. But remember, you have a free choice.

In Ezekiel, Chapter 37, God spoke to the prophet Ezekiel and told him to prophesy to dead dry bones so that they might have life. These dead bones were symbolic of the people of God, who were in a spiritually dead state.

Suddenly the joints and ligaments started to connect in the proper places. Then flesh and skin came on the bones. Although the form of life now existed, the Bible says there was no breath in these forms and therefore they were still dead. So these pretty, properly connected bones lay there lifeless. God then commanded Ezekiel to prophesy or speak to the bones again, and breath came into them. With the breath of God they stood up and created an exceedingly great army. The breath in this vision represented the Spirit of God that brought life to a dead nation.

Although every human being is connected to God, we are in a spiritually dead state without the Spirit of God. We are connected to Him by His breath, but we are alive in Him through His Spirit. This Spirit is the Holy Spirit of God, the One who was with God in the very beginning of creation, the One who *is* God and is the third person of the Trinity. God, the Father, was in heaven. God, the Son, came on earth, and God, the Holy Spirit, came from the Father to rest upon the Son and complete His work on earth.

Through the work of Jesus Christ on earth, we can have a better understanding of the purpose of God's Spirit. The Holy Spirit not only demonstrates the power of God, but also that He is a person, distinct from the Father and the Son, yet equal with them. He is God Himself, dwelling inside of believers on earth, until we go home to be with God forever in glory. In the Old Testament, God relayed messages by speaking to specific people or to His prophets.

Through the death, burial, and resurrection of Jesus Christ, the Holy Spirit is now available to all of those who believe in Him.

The Bible says He is our helper, comforter, teacher, and guide. When Jesus told His disciples that He had to leave them, He told them that He would pray for God to send them another Helper. Jesus helped them while He walked on earth, but when He ascended to heaven the Holy Spirit of God descended to help God's people who remained on earth. Jesus said in John 14:26, *"But the Helper, the Holy Spirit, whom the Father will send in my name, He will teach you all things, and bring to your remembrance all things that I said to you."*

Some people make the Spirit of God seem so difficult to understand, or make Him seem like Casper the Friendly Ghost instead of the third person of the Godhead. As a matter of fact, when I initially told Jim about the Holy Spirit being available to help him, he immediately looked at me like I was talking about a ghost. He said some people had him believe that in order to feel the Spirit of God or to hear His voice, there has to be some big explosive bang, an earthshaking experience, or a spooky event.

But God didn't send His Spirit to dwell on earth because he wanted to scare us. He knew we needed comfort and help in dealing with the many issues we face in this life. Often the Holy Spirit, who is God, speaks to our spirit with a still, small voice as He guides us and teaches us. At times the Holy Spirit will appear in a dramatic way, as He did in the upper room in the Book of Acts, Chapter 2. But I have often found Him to be that sweet comforter and guide who speaks in a quiet voice. Many times I couldn't hear Him because I was not quiet or still enough to listen to Him. I was too busy running around to listen to Him, or I was expecting a big bang and so I overlooked the signs from Him.

When Elijah prayed to God in I Kings, Chapter 19, he thought he was all alone; God wasn't in the great strong wind that tore into the mountains and broke the rocks in pieces. God was not in the earth-quake, nor was He in the fire. He answered Elijah in a still, small voice.

Just like Elijah had to listen to God in the still, small voice, I had to learn to listen to Him—and so did Jim. It didn't come overnight. In fact, Jim shared with me how just praying to God and asking Him to lead him changed his life. He learned how to depend on the presence of God's Spirit in his life, and he is now learning how to listen to that still, small voice telling him that he is not alone. He is able to listen to that voice tell him that God loves him and will never leave him. He's able to hear Him say that all things will work out for his good and that all things are possible with God.

When the Holy Spirit comes into our lives, He not only teaches us about the things of God, but He brings the characteristics of Jesus Christ with Him as described in Galatians 5:22–23. Self-control is a fruit of the Spirit or, in other words, one of the character traits of Christ that is made available to believers. We can't gain this trait on our own; that's why so many people are guilty of overindulgence in many areas of their lives. If we want the fruit of God's Spirit to be manifested in our lives, we must grow in the knowledge of God and in obedience to God. We must invite Him to have His will demonstrated in our lives.

If you want self-control, you have to allow the Spirit of God to lead you and guide you. When you find yourself overindulging and overeating, you know at that very moment that the Spirit of God is not operating in that area of your life. But when you allow Him to have control over your appetite by listening to His quiet, still voice, He can calm your raging appetite and satisfy you with his peace and presence. Galatians 5:16 reads, *"I say then: Walk in the Spirit, and you shall not fulfill the lust of the flesh."*

When you sit down and eat, bless your food, pray, and ask the Holy Spirit of God to lead you in your eating. He is right there with you, but you have to listen to Him. When you hear that voice on the inside telling you, "You know you have had enough," or "That's too much," take heed. You don't have to feel some great electrical energy flowing through your body to know He's looking out for you. God promised that every believer would be sealed with the gift of the Holy Spirit until the day of redemption (Ephesians 1:13–14), so take a deep breath, feel the Spirit, listen to His voice, and know that God is with you.

I want to share an experience that happened to me during the time I have been writing this book. The Bible says the truth shall make you free, and I was in bondage when I kept things inside, so it is my blessing to share this with you.

It's been very challenging having family obligations, being a chauffeur and a chaperon to my children, working, having ministerial responsibilities in addition to writing this book, and having other challenges (such as a recent car accident). To tell you the truth, on many days I didn't feel like exercising and would sometimes want to stop in the very beginning of my routine.

But I know for myself that the Spirit of God is real. During the times that I wanted to give up and stop, that small, inner voice of God's Spirit wouldn't let me. Even during the days when I wanted to overindulge in whatever I wanted, He spoke to my heart and would not let me.

One night after having a really busy and mentally exhausting day, I went to the twenty-four-hour grocery store at 11 P.M. to get some type of late-night snack. I wasn't even hungry; I just felt I needed something. As I walked around the store, each time I reached to pick up something, that small voice spoke to my heart and said, "No, La Vita." I walked and walked the aisles looking at everything from ice cream to cookies, cakes, and chocolate candy. As I felt the emotions of stress or the pressures of life overwhelm me, I heard something telling me to breathe. I stopped in the middle of the snack aisle and began to "feel the Spirit." As I inhaled and exhaled slowly, I concentrated on the wonderful things of God and on how He didn't bring me this far and have me overcome so many challenges in my life for me to think about giving up.

I never knew I would experience so much stress in my Christian life, but God never intended for me to take care of everything in my own life. He never intended for me to worry about anything. Because I have prayed and asked God almost daily to allow His Spirit to lead me, even during the time that I really wanted to lose the battle, He led me and I ended up buying only a bottle of water.

Remember: Don't try to do it alone.

PRAYER

Say this prayer and write it on a card to read when you are challenged:

Dear God,
Thank you for loving me so much that you never intended for me to go through this alone. I now know that you will always be with me and will never leave me. Not only that, but you have others that I can share with as we support one another in brotherly love. I ask that your Holy Spirit leads me to the right fitness partner. I also ask that you help me learn how to recognize that quiet, still voice of Your Spirit as He guides my eating and exercise habits (and in every other area in my life). Remove any pride or shame that could hinder my progress. I want to be free from neglecting my body; I want to be healthy, and I want you to freely use me to be a blessing to others. In Jesus' name I pray. Amen

Study Scriptures

JOSHUA 1:9
Have I not commanded you? Be strong and of good courage; do not be afraid, nor be dismayed, for the Lord your God is with you wherever you go.

JOHN 14:26

But the Helper, the Holy Spirit, whom the Father will send in My name, He will teach you all things and bring to your remembrance all things that I said to you.

PHILIPPIANS 2:3–4

Let nothing be done through selfish ambition or conceit, but in lowliness of mind let each esteem others better than himself. Let each of you look out not only for your own interests, but also for the interests of others.

ACTIVITIES

1. Pray and ask God to lead you to the right person or people for support. Whether it's your fitness partner, your prayer partner, a personal trainer, or family members or friends, begin to develop a support system for those times you won't feel like living healthy or may need encouragement.

2. Find someone—other than your support—whom you can help. God created us to help one another. You don't have to wait until the battle is over to share with others. Just be honest with yourself. It may be difficult in the beginning, but as you trust God and begin to rely on His guidance you'll begin to experience the joy in victory. You could be the very tool God uses to make others more aware of the importance of healthy living and to encourage them to do the same.

3. Feel the Spirit. Choose at least three times during the day when you can practice this activity. Sit down and relax in a quiet location. Inhale and exhale slowly three times as you clear your mind of all of your problems, concerns, and thoughts of the day. Begin to focus on the things of God: how He said He will always be with you; how He's able to help you overcome any obstacle; how much He loves you and how His desire is for you to live an abundant, healthy life. Then ask God to allow His Holy Spirit to minister to your heart. Tell Him that you want to get to know His voice.

You may want to practice this throughout the week. It is a great way to prepare for war during a time of peace. Then, when you feel the urge to overindulge or get another helping you know you don't need, immediately inhale and exhale slowly; because you've practiced and trained your mind to focus on the things of God after the breaths, you should begin to clear your mind of whatever is sparking your desire to overindulge. You can listen to the still voice of God's Spirit letting you know that you have had enough.

Get rid of the excuses that stop you from being "fit for God"

1. CRAVINGS

Cravings are normal, but if you often experience uncontrollable cravings, it may be your spirit and not your body crying out for food. Allow God to fill you by seeking to develop a personal relationship with Him through His Word and prayer. **Proverbs 13:25** *The righteous eats to the satisfying of the soul, but the stomach of the wicked shall be in want.*

2. ENVY

Having envy for others only causes you harm. Be glad for what God has done for others and maybe you will get your breakthrough. **Proverbs 14:30** *A sound heart is life to the body, but envy is rottenness to the bones.*

3. GLUTTONY

The Bible speaks of the glutton and the drunkard in the same sentence. Gluttony can have the same effect as alcohol by increasing your risk for illness and making you sluggish and unable to function at your best. When you want to overeat and you know you've had enough, do what it takes—stop, pray, drink some water, or just put on your Reeboks and run. **Proverbs 23:20–21** *Do not mix with wine bibbers or with gluttonous eaters of meat; for the drunkard and the glutton will come to poverty, and drowsiness will clothe a man with rags.*

4. STRESS

The Bible says there is a time for everything. The problem is we try to do too much at one time. Allow God to help you use your time wisely and guide you to do what is necessary in the appropriate time. **Ecclesiastes 3:1** *For everything there is a season, a time for every purpose under heaven.*

5. NEGATIVE THOUGHTS

If your thought life is hindering you from being all that God has created you to be, your mind is on the wrong thing. Get your mind in order and your body will follow. **II Corinthians 10:4–5** *For the weapons of our warfare are not carnal but mighty in God for the pulling down of strongholds, casting down arguments and every high thing that exalts itself against the knowledge of God, bringing every thought into captivity to the obedience of Christ.*

6. LACK OF FORGIVENESS

Forgiving others is not an option. Jesus commanded it. When you don't forgive others, not only are you held in bondage and unable to enjoy the freedom of perfect peace, but God cannot forgive you for your sins. **Matthew 6:14–15** *For if you forgive men their trespasses, your heavenly Father will also forgive you. But if you do not forgive men their trespasses, neither will your Father forgive your trespasses.*

7. UNHAPPINESS

If you are unhappy, maybe you need to evaluate who or what you are putting your trust in. Trusting the Almighty God to have control of your life can only lead you to happiness. **Proverbs 16:20** *He who heeds the word wisely will find good. And whoever trusts in the Lord, happy is he.*

8. FEELING UNLOVED

It's human nature to want to be loved. Many people have experienced many disappointments because they have looked for love in all the wrong places. Many have discovered what they thought was love wasn't love at all. But God's love is not based on what you do, what you say, where you live, how much money you make, or how great a figure you have. He loves you unconditionally. Others can take their love away, but nothing can separate you from the love of God. **Romans 8:38–39** *For I am persuaded that neither death nor life, nor angels nor principalities nor powers, nor things present nor things to come, nor height nor depth, nor any other created thing, shall be able to separate us from the love of God which is in Christ Jesus our Lord.*

Week Seven

Rest Your Body, Mind, and Spirit

... And He Rested on the Seventh Day from All His Work
Which He Had Done.

—GENESIS 2:2

Two clients taught me the importance of rest, a factor in fitness that I had not seriously considered in the past. The clients, whom I'll call Erica and JoAnn, had a lot in common. They were both full-time registered nurses in their thirties with small children and demanding jobs. Erica was a single mother and JoAnn was married.

Yet Erica, with more responsibility and no one to help her, was energetic, pleasant, and positive. JoAnn was always tired and complaining about having to work and take care of small children. There were times when I didn't look forward to meeting with JoAnn because I knew she was going to complain nonstop. She had a supportive husband who worked hard, paid the majority of the bills, and gave her the option of working part-time and going back to school. Regardless, whenever I saw her she had another sad story. She brushed it off, saying it was just her personality to be easily irritated and frustrated.

I don't believe people have to be miserable, irritable, and tired most of the time. I was also raising small children and had to work full-time.

JoAnn wanted me to help her tone her body. We discussed eating right and exercising, but I felt I was missing something. I was still a new fitness consultant and I had a lot to learn. I was running with Erica one day when it dawned on me what was wrong with JoAnn. Erica was full of life, as usual, and her aerobic conditioning was improving. Listening to her lively conversation made running several miles around the track seem like only one mile. She spoke about her job, the different patients she encountered, and how mentally and physically draining the job could be, especially since she then had to come home and care for her children.

"What gives you the motivation to do everything you need to do?" I asked.

"Thank God I exercise, eat right, and make sure I get my rest," she said. "I don't let anyone stop me from getting my rest because I can't function well without it."

She said without sufficient sleep she felt sluggish and irritable and couldn't deal with the kids or patients, couldn't concentrate well, and sometimes even felt depressed. When the kids went to bed, she turned off the phone and turned on the answering machine so she could relax.

That was it! Rest was the missing something in JoAnn's life. When I met with JoAnn again, the first thing I asked was "How much rest do you get?"

"Very little," she answered.

And while Erica avoided drinking coffee all day, JoAnn started off her day with a cup of coffee and sipped the brew throughout the day to keep her going.

God is truly an awesome planner and Creator. The Bible says God created the heavens and the earth in six days. Then on the seventh day God rested from all of His work. Did God actually need rest? Did God need to sit down and take a lunch break, or get a catnap or a good night's sleep like you and I? No, God is spirit; He is eternal and doesn't have a physical body like you and I have.

Psalm 121 even says God neither sleeps nor slumbers. So why did God rest? The Bible says God rested because His work was now complete. The number seven, the day that God rested, is the number in the Bible used to indicate completeness or perfection. I also believe one of the reasons He rested was to set an example before humankind. He created the earth in six days and rested on the seventh, so we observe a seven-day week. He sanctified the seventh day and made it holy, and we recognize the Sabbath as a holy day. (However, in Christianity we don't observe the Sabbath on the seventh day, as in the Jewish tradition; we observe it on the first day of the week in recognition of the resurrection of Jesus Christ.)

God demonstrated that rest is an important part of humankind's existence by first putting it into practice Himself. When God delivered the children of Israel out of the land of Egypt, not only did He satisfy their need for food and water, but He also provided them with rest. God told the children of Israel for six days they would gather the manna sent down from heaven, but on the seventh day they would cease from all their work. He also told them that even their ox and donkey, their servants, and strangers should rest on the seventh day. Even when God led the children of Israel into the wilderness by the cloud, He gave them rest from their journey. Wherever the cloud stopped, they set up their tents and rested until the cloud moved. They moved with the cloud, but they also rested with the cloud.

Jesus Christ was on a specific mission for God. As a matter of fact, He was on the most important assignment for the human race, yet He told his disciples in Mark 6:31, *"Come aside by yourselves to a deserted place and rest a while."* Jesus' disciples were probably so excited about the great things they were doing with the Lord that if

Jesus had not told them to rest, they never would have stopped. Jesus confirmed with the Father the importance of rest for the body.

God knew that in the hustle and bustle of our society we would get so caught up in the everyday affairs of living we would forget a basic need such as rest. And He was right. Many people today complain of fatigue and exhaustion, and of not having enough time to do everything they need to do. Others rely on coffee and other stimulants to push them beyond their body's limit. Many health problems of today are associated with fatigue and overwork—some people are called workaholics. We insist that we don't have enough hours in the day to do everything we need to do, insinuating that the Omnipotent, Almighty, Wise, and Eternal Creator somehow didn't know what He was doing when He created the twenty-four-hour day. God never intended for us to get so caught up in money, success, and doing so much that we forget about what is really important in life. If we truly needed more time, He would have given it to us. The problem is not that we don't have enough time; the problem is that we don't use our time wisely. We try to do too much or we waste precious time.

God Himself set the stage by being an example. The Sabbath was a day set aside when the children of Israel could reflect on the goodness of God, on who He is and all He has done for them. The word "Sabbath" comes from the Hebrew word meaning "to cease." When they were in the wilderness, the children of Israel gathered twice as much manna on the sixth day so there would be enough for them to rest on the seventh day. Later, the Jewish household cooked the previous day so that on the Sabbath they could focus on God and rest from their daily work. Even their animals rested every seven days. The Sabbath was so important that God gave it to Moses as one of the Ten Commandments and it became a law. Breaking this law resulted in a death sentence.

When God spoke to Moses and gave him the Sabbath Law for

the children of Israel in Exodus 31:16, He said that the children of Israel shall keep the Sabbath and observe it throughout all of their generations. Then He says in verse 17, *"It is a sign between me and the children of Israel forever; for in six days the Lord made the heavens and the earth and on the seventh day He rested and was refreshed."*

When God designed the human body, He designed it to need rest. Without this rest it is impossible to function properly and continue to grow. If you have a cat or dog, I am sure you have seen your pet rest. There are even times when fish appear to be more still than at other times. If you watch some of the nature programs, you'll see that lions and tigers seem to always be resting. Even the earth rests with different seasons as the soil, plants, flowers, and trees bloom or become more productive. We see the importance of rest for humans in newborn babies, who spend most of their hours asleep, briefly waking for food, then returning back to sleep. Adults may not require as much sleep as young children, but rest is still vital for our total well-being.

When you hear the word "rest," you may automatically think about leisure or sleep. But during this step, I'm going to discuss three types of rest to satisfy the need of the total person, body, mind, and spirit.

PHYSICAL REST

As human beings, we are the only creatures that push ourselves until we are physically and emotionally exhausted. I guess that's the consequence of being "intelligent" creatures. We think we have so much to do and not enough time to do it, so we try to make up for the extra time by robbing our bodies of the refreshment that sleep provides. This happens especially in American culture; other cultures often take longer lunch hours and even shut down the town for hours in the afternoon so that people can stop to rest and relax.

We do quite the opposite. Many of us work right through our lunch hours and try to cram as many activities as possible into the day until we finally pass out in bed from exhaustion.

Total well-being and weight management involve not only eating right and exercising, but also getting sufficient sleep and rest for the body. Our bodies are not like computers or machines that you turn on and keep running until you decide to turn them off. The human body will break down if you run it without rest, and this may be shown through irritability, anxiety, stress, the inability to concentrate, frustration, illnesses, or even depression.

Before I paid attention to my body, I always ran myself ragged until I got sick. If I don't get enough rest, I become forgetful and may even start nodding off to sleep while I'm driving. Being tired also affects your reaction time, which is why we often hear reports about insufficient rest being a concern for truck drivers traveling the highways.

Remember Elijah in I Kings, Chapter 19? He was the prophet of God who felt so all alone that he asked God if he could die. Well, Elijah also had another problem. After he ran an entire day's journey in the desert, he was exhausted, discouraged, and depressed. The angel of the Lord told him to get up and eat and drink something. After he did this, he rested. He then got up a second time, ate and drank again, and rested again. He was then strengthened and continued his forty-day journey. Although Elijah was miraculously used by the Spirit of God, he was still in a physical body with physical restrictions and limitations. He needed the food for strength, and he also needed the rest to refresh his body and prepare him to continue his journey ahead.

There is no doubt that not getting sufficient sleep is bad for your health. When most people are extremely tired, they tend to overeat. Have you ever found yourself staying up late and snacking on everything you could find? I know I felt that somehow the snacking helped me to stay awake when I was up late working or studying.

So how much sleep is enough? It is estimated that you need between seven and eight hours daily. But this is only an estimate. The actual amount varies from person to person. What is important is that you listen to your body to determine the amount of sleep that is right for you. Develop a personal rhythm by allowing the sleep to occur around the same time each day and for a constant number of hours. There will be times when, for whatever reason, you will not get much sleep. But losing a night's sleep or a few hours' sleep is not detrimental to your health.

Just as you should listen to your body to avoid overeating, you must listen to your body to determine whether or not you are getting sufficient rest. Do you wake up refreshed and feeling renewed, ready for the new day? Or do you wake up still groggy and tired? Do you wake up naturally on your own or do you hit the snooze button several times before you get up? Or like JoAnn and many of her coworkers, do you rely on a caffeinated beverage such as coffee to get you going and keep you going? Do you allow your body to naturally signal you when it's time to slow down? Remember: Insufficient sleep can make you feel physically drained and affect your overall mood and attitude, your ability to function at your best.

On the other hand, too much sleep is not better than just enough. Proverbs 6:9–11 reads, *"How long will you slumber, O sluggard? When will you rise from your sleep? A little sleep, a little slumber, a little folding of the hands to sleep—so shall your poverty come on you like a prowler, and your need like an armed man."*

This Scripture warns against getting too much sleep, which can create laziness. Have you ever slept longer than usual and found yourself still tired? I know from personal experience that if I get too much sleep, I'm tired and unable to have a productive day. As mentioned in Exodus 23:12 and 34:21, we need to set aside the right amount of time for sufficient rest.

Find out what works for you and be consistent with your sleeping pattern. For instance, if you normally get six hours of sleep and you notice you are always tired, then that is a good indication that you need more rest. See how you feel if you extend your sleep by going to bed earlier or setting the alarm for later. If you normally sleep nine hours and you are still tired (and you don't have any medical conditions), that is a good sign you are getting too much sleep. I think most adults know what really works for them. It is just a matter of listening to your body and not masking what your body is saying by taking stimulants to keep going.

The amount of sleep you require may change at different times of your life. For instance, if you start a new exercise program, you may need more rest in the beginning because your body needs more recovery time from physical activity. Once you become better physically conditioned and your body adapts, it will require less recovery time and therefore need less sleep.

Let me repeat: God did not make any mistakes. He created a twenty-four-hour day and a human body that can get sufficient rest within that period of time. Actually, I think if it weren't for Thomas Edison and the fact that we now have electricity, we would probably get more rest because we wouldn't be able to spend late nights at the office or stay up working or studying until the wee hours in the morning. At one time people rose at sunrise and went to bed at sunset. Although times have drastically changed, the human body is still made of the same flesh it was years ago and still needs to be rejuvenated and revived with sufficient rest. Remember, what is important is the total amount of sleep you get, the quality of sleep, and that your sleep is continuous—not broken up with constant awakenings or interruptions. Here are some tips so you can have a sweet sleep as the psalmist wrote in Psalm 3:24:

1. Eat healthier. A general rule of thumb I like to use is "If God didn't make it, eat it sparingly." Many foods that are not natural are processed such that the nutrients have been removed and other additives and artificial ingredients added. Avoid these foods, which can be taxing to your digestive system, making it work harder or making it sluggish, which in turn affects your sleep.

2. Avoid eating late at night. Not only can eating heavy meals at night add on the extra calories and pounds, but high-calorie, high-fat foods make your digestive system work harder, which may wake you up in the middle of the night or keep you awake. A heavy meal before bedtime is a sure way to get a bad night's sleep.

3. Exercise regularly. Exercise can help relieve the stress, anxiety, and tension that may prevent you from sleeping well. It can also tire out your body to help you sleep well.

4. Wind down before you go to bed. You can wind down by listening to soft, relaxing music, by reading something peaceful, by taking a warm, soothing bubble bath, or by watching a peaceful television program.

5. Reduce your intake of caffeine. Although health experts don't recommend that you give up coffee and other caffeinated beverages altogether, you should consume them with caution and cut back if you consume too much. Consuming more than 200 milligrams of caffeine a day (the amount of two cups of coffee or three colas) can be addictive and affect your ability to sleep, according to health experts. Consider stopping your caffeine intake by midafternoon at the latest to give your body a chance to wind down.

MENTAL REST

You may find yourself physically exhausted and ready to just crash, but unable to rest. Or you may get sufficient rest for the body and still find you are tired and drained. This can be because your mind may be racing, thinking about the events of the day or the multitude of things you need to do the next day. Although you could be sitting down, resting the body, the mind could be working away, thinking and trying to figure out important decisions and solutions. It's important to get enough rest for the mind, also.

The mind is so powerful that people have spoken their own destiny—positive or negative—into existence. Everything in your physical surroundings can be fine, but you may still be stressed or depressed because of what is going on in your mind. Some people have physical symptoms of an illness or pain because of the thoughts in their mind. I feel that most of our so-called problems are associated with the mind rather than physical circumstances.

JoAnn and Erica were a perfect example of this. Although they had similar jobs and small children, Erica found the time to get sufficient rest and peace for her mind; therefore, she had a more pleasant outlook and a positive attitude. JoAnn had help with her children and household responsibilities, yet she always complained and was often easily irritated. Even when JoAnn began to eat right and exercise, she was still a rather frustrated person. We discussed her possible need for more rest and she committed to getting enough sleep. She turned off her ringer on her phone at a certain time at night to make sure she got uninterrupted sleep.

JoAnn now had the time to get enough sleep but she often found herself tossing and turning, waking up several times in the middle of the night. Although it can be normal to wake up several times during the night to change your sleeping position, JoAnn's awakenings were more than just turning over from her back to her side.

At first I thought maybe she was having marital problems, but I didn't feel that I was in a position to ask her that. As I listened to her more and more, I discovered that she saw problems in things that were not problems for most people. She talked about what she should be doing and what she should have done, or what she needed to do. During our conversations she often moved quickly from one topic of concern to another, whether it was about her weight, how much she paid for child care, or wanting new hours at work. Although she needed rest for her body, it was obvious that she also needed sufficient rest and peace for her mind.

I could relate to JoAnn because I remembered my mental state when I struggled with overeating, depression, and insomnia. When I began to pursue some of the goals and opportunities I thought I had missed in life, my physical circumstances dramatically improved but I didn't have peace and rest in my mind. I felt tremendous stress and anxiety and often found myself totally exhausted even when I didn't exert much energy; or I'd find myself lying in bed looking up at the ceiling, unable to sleep. I worried about everything because I always expected the worst.

Matthew 6:25 reads, *"Therefore I say to you, do not worry about your life, what you will eat or what you will drink; nor about your body, what you will put on. Is not life more than food and the body more than clothing?"*

I read this Scripture one night when I was up late one night having a snack—and an anxiety—attack. It was as though God was letting me know that He knew about all of my concerns, but He didn't want me to worry about them. At this point it wasn't about what I was eating, but it was about what was eating me. I realized that worry didn't accomplish anything, but caused harm to my mind and eventually my body through overindulging. I had to learn how to deal with the present day and trust God to continue to meet my daily needs.

It's still challenging sometimes as I'm faced with new situations. But I've come a long way by learning how to put some biblical principles into practice. So what do you do when your mind is racing faster than you can keep up with it and you feel overwhelmed with the cares of life? How do you slow down and rest your mind? Let's look at a couple of passages in the Bible regarding rest.

King David, a psalmist, a mighty man of God and one of the greatest kings in the history of mankind, spoke of rest in Psalm 23, one of the most popularly read Psalms in the Bible. Verses 1 and 2 read, *"The Lord is my shepherd; I shall not want. He makes me lie down in green pastures; He leads me beside the still waters."* In this Psalm, David compares God's provision for His children to the protection and care a shepherd provides for his flock. David spent many years as a shepherd, so he was writing from his own personal experience. In biblical days shepherds lived hard lives, for they stayed with their sheep to protect them. Sheep without a shepherd are vulnerable and their very lives can be in danger. But as long as they follow the guidance of the shepherd, he protects them and cares for them with his very life.

Not only does a shepherd protect the flock and provide for all of its needs (verse 1), but the shepherd also leads the flock to a quiet place, a place of rest, peace, and safety (verse 2). Likewise, when we follow the directions of God, who is ultimately our Good Shepherd, we, too, can experience that quiet place where contentment and peace for our minds is possible.

In the beginning of creation, God gives us another example to follow. The Bible says He saw everything He created and indeed it was *very good*, and He rested on the seventh day. Part of God's rest included reflection on what He had done. He knew that it was a magnificent work.

Do you always worry about the future? Do you always have negative thoughts about what you need to do or what you should have done? Do you spend time reflecting on the positive accomplishments in your life or do you spend most of your time focusing on the *bad*? After each step of creation, God did not say what He needed to do next. He did not call the chaotic state of the universe or the darkness "bad."

He simply did something about it, enjoyed its completion, reflected on how good it was, and then He moved on to the next step.

I truly believe God stopped to reflect on his work so that we would take note of the importance of rest for our sanity. Remember, God had the power to just zap the entire universe and all life forms into existence simultaneously. But He didn't. He specifically recorded His steps of creation in the Bible. He knew that eventually we would live in a world in which we are overwhelmed with the hustle and bustle of everyday living rather than focusing on what really matters in life. He knew that we would need an example to let us know it is not His intention for His creation to be consumed with mental concerns and the stress of daily living. Therefore, He demonstrated the importance of appreciating what we have accomplished or what is positive in our lives.

By reflecting, you look back on what you have done and appreciate it. In regard to weight loss, even if you do not see the physical results right away, taking any step in the right direction is an accomplishment. Can you appreciate the fact that you bought this book because you have the desire to live healthier? Can you look back and appreciate how you feel more motivated to do it God's way this time? Can you appreciate the fact that you are not giving up? And you may have started making physical changes such as thinking more positively, drinking more water, eating more natural foods, or just exercising. Can you reflect on the positive changes that are taking place in your life and health today?

You cannot be concerned or consumed with what needs to be done tomorrow, next week, or next month. You cannot even be consumed with whether you are losing weight fast enough or what areas you find the most difficult to overcome. Even if you feel you have made mistakes, you can look back and evaluate them to learn how not to make those mistakes again. Likewise, we can learn from our accomplishments.

David, who was referred to as a man after God's own heart, knew the importance of reflection when faced with battles and great challenges in life. When he came up against the giant Goliath in I Samuel 17:31–52, it looked humanly impossible for him to defeat a nine-foot-nine-inch-tall giant covered in armor from head to foot. Goliath also had a shield and a sword, and the young David only had a sling and three smooth pebbles. This situation looked so impossible that David's own brothers mocked him.

But reflection can be a powerful tool, especially when you are faced with great challenges. Although many criticized him, David didn't allow that to discourage him. He told King Saul that God had delivered him from bears and lions when he protected his father's sheep, and the same God would surely deliver him from this Philistine. David didn't look at how big the problem was or how impossible it seemed. He looked back and remembered what God had already done for him. He kept his eye on the ability of God and was able to miraculously defeat this giant with only a sling and a pebble.

David could have viewed his battle with Goliath as a big problem, as King Saul and the entire army of Israel did. But David knew better. Just think how much easier our lives would be if we adopted David's wonderful perspective when faced with challenges.

Remember this as you work your way through the Fit for God program. If your only improvement is that you are now drinking four cups of water, compared to drinking none before you started the program, appreciate your accomplishment. Don't worry about tomorrow, and continue to allow the Shepherd to lead you to the place where you will have abundant rest and peace in Him.

Apostle Paul gives another example of how you can put your mind at rest in the book of Philippians, Chapter 4. He starts out in Philippians 4:6 saying be anxious for nothing, but take everything to God in prayer; then you will have peace for your heart and your mind. He concludes in verse 8 saying, *"Finally brethren, whatever things are true, whatever things are noble, whatever things are just, whatever things are pure, whatever things are lovely, whatever things are of good report, if there is any virtue and if there is anything praiseworthy—meditate on these things."*

The thoughts in your mind can affect your whole outlook and your behavior. Paul, although a prisoner awaiting trial, tells how to have rest for your mind by meditating on those things that are true, noble, just, pure, lovely, of good report, virtuous, and praiseworthy.

Have you taken the time today to meditate on the things that are worth praising God for? Have you meditated on the fact that God created you with a purpose in mind? How about the fact that you are special to God and He loves you unconditionally? Have you meditated on the fact that in spite of what you have gone through, you have a sound mind? Have you meditated on the fact that God has given you another chance today, when many others didn't wake up this morning? There is so much to be thankful for. It may take some practice to learn how to meditate on those wonderful things of God. But just as with everything else, the more you do it, the easier it will become.

You want to be just as careful about your mental intake as you are with your food intake. What type of negative influences do you put in your mind? Do you often think about the negative? The wrong kinds of television programs, books, music, and conversations can fill your mind with negative thoughts that adversely affect your life. This can manifest in your actions and your attitude as well. Take all your concerns to God in prayer, think on those lovely things and the goodness of God, and allow Him to fill your mind with His perfect peace and rest.

Although we should remember God daily, we should especially on the Sabbath because it also allowed God's children to be refreshed and renewed. Jesus Christ said that the Sabbath was made for man. This confirms that God was setting an example for us in Genesis.

Although in the Christian faith we celebrate the resurrection of Christ by worshiping on Sundays, it can be a far cry from Sabbath rest. This Sabbath rest should be a time of refreshment, a time of renewal, a time of connecting mentally and spiritually with our Creator to find inner peace and tranquility; and a time for meditating on His goodness, His mercy, and His grace. However, our daily routines as well as some of our church schedules are filled with hectic appointments, engagements, and events.

Many people come to the house of God for Sabbath rest still in their overbooked routines. Especially in ministry, it is so easy to get so busy preparing for certain programs and church services that the Sabbath rest never occurs. I love the house of God and God's people. But the true focus of Christianity can easily be lost with all the routines and what many people perceive as "working for the Lord."

The truth is: God doesn't really need our work. God is almighty; He created the universe and all that's in it. He can raise up an entire congregation out of rocks if He wants to, or He can use the angels and they can do a better and quicker job than we can. What God really wants is for us to acknowledge Him, trust Him, and follow His directives for our lives. Do you take the time to focus on God? Do you go to church as a routine, or do you go to find refreshment and renewal through Him? Do you fellowship at all?

God tells us in the Bible that fellowship with other believers is very important and we should not forsake it (Hebrews 10:25). But God also makes it clear that we need to take the time to specifically focus on Him. I believe that if you are involved in the church and find yourself too busy on Sundays with responsibilities or commitments in the church, you can choose another day of the week to dedicate completely to God. Setting aside the time to acknowledge God, to reflect on what He has already done and to meditate on what he will continue to do in your life is the greatest way to put your mind at rest in a world full of disarray and distress.

SPIRITUAL REST

Study God's Word

Although physical rest is needed for the body and mental rest is needed for the mind, there is a deeper rest needed by humankind that is beyond human comprehension. It is as though each human being is on a journey, searching for something far greater than weight loss, a good night's sleep, or tranquility for the mind. It is a journey to satisfy an inner uneasiness that cannot be easily put to rest. Although many of us try to resolve these feelings by striving for more education, more money, more power, or a higher position, this uneasiness still exists.

It appears to be human nature to want to accumulate as much as possible. Yet people still find themselves not satisfied—not having peace, or rest, in their lives. Those who don't have a lot of money think that money will resolve these feelings. They find themselves obsessed with seeking more and more, but they never feel fulfilled. Others find themselves in debt from living beyond their financial means, trying to fill that void.

There is an inner hunger that must be fed. People try to feed it in all kinds of ways, which can manifest in drug addiction, alcoholism, sex addiction, and overeating. Food seems to be the safest way for many people—myself included—to try to satisfy this hunger.

But this hunger goes beyond cravings and sensual desires. Even when these fleshly desires have been temporarily fulfilled, there is still an aching and a need for permanent satisfaction.

JoAnn seemingly had no real reason to worry, yet she often found herself tossing and turning in bed at night. She had a good career, a supportive husband, no financial difficulties, and two beautiful girls. Yet she was frustrated often and easily agitated. She eventually went back to school and got a new job. Her husband bought her a new car, she had more help with the kids, but there was still something missing that manifested itself in her disposition and her preoccupation with food. Even after she began to care for her health by eating healthier and by exercising and trying to get sufficient rest, she still found herself carousing through the refrigerator and eating out of control at times.

Does it ever seem that nothing satisfies you? Can you relate to JoAnn's story? Or maybe you feel your life would be better if you were in JoAnn's shoes?

Although I am an ordained minister and a personal trainer, I had a client named Marcus who I concluded needed more than I could offer. It was one of the few times when I wanted to give up on a client.

Marcus was overweight and had high blood pressure. He started his workout program, but he lived to eat. He didn't drink alcohol, smoke, or do any drugs. His bad habit was a ferocious appetite. I had the opportunity to see him eat during a business lunch before he became a client. He chowed down each slice of bread in two bites, then asked the waitress to bring another basket of bread. He had a salad saturated with dressing, a bowl of soup, soda refills, and the main entrée, which included a juicy, medium-rare steak. He cleaned his plates and emptied the bread basket. He got his dessert to go. I thought, "My God, where do I start?"

As time progressed, I noticed other things about Marcus. He was obsessed with making more and more money, yet was never satisfied with anything. He was in his third marriage and had many sexual relationships before and in between marriages.

I eventually worked with Marcus and his wife together. Marcus said his wife was the problem in their marriage; that his ex-wives also did him wrong, and his mother and father caused him grief, too. He blamed everybody else for his problems. One time right in front of me he told his wife that she was the reason he was overweight because she didn't exercise enough with him. He even blamed her for his anger problems, saying she didn't know when to shut up. His wife was at the point where she didn't want to talk to him about anything because he was a time bomb waiting to explode. She said he misconstrued whatever she said. She was hesitant to go out with him in public because anything could set him off and she didn't want to be embarrassed. Their children had also witnessed his temper tantrums. When she expressed concern for his health because of his extra weight and asked him to get a physical to make sure he was okay, he exploded and yelled, "Oh, so now you don't like your big fat husband!"

I had to take off my hat to his wife and his ex-wives. I thought to myself that even as a minister, it would take supernatural help or the hand of God Himself to help me if I had to deal with this type of man in a personal relationship. Then I began to feel sorry for him. Something inside him was screaming out for help. He was always trying to find something, or someone, to satisfy this internal yearning.

Marcus and JoAnn had different circumstances, but it was as though a raging sea was inside both of them, waiting to be calmed and put to rest.

We have to go back to the beginning to understand why human beings can experience an internal void that may be manifested as a preoccupation with security, physical desires, or finding no real rest or satisfaction. We have to go back to the beginning to understand what it is in some people that is screaming out for help.

The Bible says humankind is unique. Man was made in the image of God. We are made in His image to be rational and intellectual beings, and we are also created with a tripartite nature, one consisting of more than just a body—with a spirit and a soul as well. When God blew breath into man's nostrils, He released a part of Himself into each human being.

This precious life resource is a gift from God given to every living being.

So where is the spirit of man? It is still inside of each and every human being. It is still longing to commune with the Creator. The spirit of man is not at peace as it searches for the fulfillment to put the hunger pangs at rest. It is on a continuing journey, crying out through the body and mind, expressing its desire to connect back with God through physical appetites, mental distress, and an inability to be satisfied with anything.

Both JoAnn and Marcus discovered that their problem was not a physical problem but a spiritual problem. How could they satisfy the inner desire that plagued their very existence? Many Christians would likely answer this question by saying, "They need to accept Jesus as Savior." However, both had accepted Jesus as Savior and still had these problems. I was able to help both of them because I'd had a similar problem.

I had accepted Christ as my Savior and still found myself obsessed with food, never satisfied, and eventually traveling down a dark tunnel of despair and depression. After many years of anxiety attacks, tears, bingeing, and eventually making an appointment to see a psychiatrist, I decided to pursue rest and peace for my soul. I discovered that in order to put the spirit at ease, saying that you are a Christian, toting a Bible, wearing a "Jesus" T-shirt, wearing a cross, or having a bumper sticker is not enough. Man's spirit needs to be connected back to God in order to be truly satisfied.

Let's look at these Scriptures:

PSALM 42:1–2

As the deer pants for the water brooks, so pants my soul for You, O God. My soul thirsts for God, for the living God.

PSALM 63:1

O God, You are my God; early will I seek You; my flesh longs for You;
in a dry and thirsty land where there is no water.

PSALM 84:2

My heart and flesh cry out for the living God.

The psalmists learned that the crying out in their body and soul
was not for materialistic gain, wealth, sex, or food. Many of them
discovered this after they tried everything they could, and these little "gods" (wealth, things, people, food, and drink) still could not
satisfy that deep, inner longing. They discovered that this panting of
the soul, this thirst in their inner man, this longing and crying out
of even the flesh was a yearning to have a personal connection with
the one and only God that has the gift of life. This yearning could
be satisfied only by having a personal relationship with God and by
being in His presence, which is the fullness of joy (Psalm 16:11).

Just like JoAnn and Marcus, I was tired of my belly being my
"god." Philippians 3:19 reads, "*. . . whose end is destruction, whose*
god is their belly, and whose glory is in their shame—who set their
mind on earthly things."

I didn't want to continue being a slave to my appetite and living
a lie. Behind closed doors I ate myself into a state of intoxication. I
was tired of food affecting my mood. My belly was leading me to destruction. And as much as I hated to admit it, the Bible tells me that
I was a glutton. The Bible says that gluttony can lead to laziness and
poverty, and that anyone who is a companion of gluttony shames his
father (Proverbs 23:21 and 28:7; Titus 1:12).

Gluttony is a sin because it destroys the temple of the living God.
The Bible states that the least we can do for God is present our bodies as a living sacrifice to Him (Romans 12:1). I needed help; I
couldn't do it alone.

So I decided to take my sister LaReese's advice and do whatever it took to develop a personal relationship with the living God. I had heard about Him and read about Him; now it was time to get to know Him.

I needed to find rest for my inner man. I learned that just as my body needs food for strength and rest for refreshment, my inner man needs spiritual food to put its hunger pangs at rest. I found a rest much deeper than that needed by my body or my mind. This rest came from the Word of God and from prayer.

When people ask me how I overcame bingeing, depression, and anxiety, and also lost the weight, my first response is "Through the Word of God." Then they normally ask, "How did you really do it? Didn't you have to change your diet and exercise?"

Of course I did, but that was not enough. It wasn't until I committed to reading God's Word that a permanent change began to take place.

I cannot express how important it is to read the Word of God for yourself. I've discovered that many Christians do not read the Bible regularly. A Christian without the Word is like a fish out of water. You'll flip and flop back and forth until you finally die, spiritually that is. When God told Joshua in Chapter 1 of the Book of Joshua that it was time to go and conquer the Promised Land, He also told him what would be the key to his success.

Take a look at Joshua 1:8: *"This Book of the Law shall not depart from your mouth, but you shall meditate in it day and night, that you may observe to do according to all that is written in it. For then you will make your way prosperous and then you will have good success."*

The Book of the Law in those days was God's Word. Although many war heroes may be impressed with the nation of Israel's military strategy in conquering the land, God told Joshua the real strategy for success and prosperity. He told Joshua to read and study the Book of the Law; then He also told him not only to meditate on it (think about it over and over), but to do what it says. The Book of the Law gained the Israelites success in conquering the Promised Land, and reading the Bible helped with my success in losing the weight and keeping it off.

What exactly is the Word of God or the Bible? The Bible *is* the inspired Word of God. The Greek word for "inspired" literally means "God-breathed" in English (II Timothy 3:16). God actually breathed his Word into men so they could write the truths of God. The writers wrote by the guiding and the authority of the Holy Spirit of God. It makes sense to me that the Word is "God-breathed" because every time I read the Bible it's as though God Himself is connecting with my spirit, giving me whatever I need to put my spirit at rest.

In addition to getting the proper knowledge to care for my body, I learned that the proper knowledge to care for all of me was found only in the Bible. As we read in Joshua 1:8, the Word can help you prosper and give you success; it can also light your path (Psalm 119:105), heal you (Psalm 107:20), bless you abundantly (Psalm 1:1–2 and Deuteronomy 28:1–14), and satisfy your inner hunger (Matthew 4:4). The Word of God can help you understand more about God and how much He loves you, and let you know that He is there to help you and guide you in every situation.

As I mentioned earlier, Marcus is one client I really wanted to stop training. He had a very strong, stubborn, controlling personality, and although he knew nothing about fitness, he tried to control the training. I personally felt that I didn't have to tolerate it. But thank God for God's spirit in me, because I knew that while I could not help Marcus, God could. I shared certain Scriptures with him and was finally able to encourage him to read God's Word for Himself. His wife couldn't change him, and it wasn't my job to change him, but the Word of God was more powerful than his set ways. It was as though the Word provided him with a mirror in which he could look and examine himself. He realized he expected too much from other people and that he needed to rely on God—

not his little "god," his belly—to fill his void. He also realized he was responsible for his own behavior, and that he didn't have the right to mistreat or blame other people for his problems. He was deeply sorry for the pain he had caused his wife and children, and he realized he needed to continue to develop a personal relationship with God for his continued healing, strength, and spiritual growth.

JoAnn came to appreciate the wonderful life she had and realized that what was missing was her spiritual connection to God. It also helped her control her late-night snack attacks by soothing her emotions and spirit. Marcus's change was gradual but incredible, because with God all things are possible.

The Word of God uplifted me when I was down and out; it encouraged me, gave me hope, renewed my mind, and strengthened my soul. It comforted me during times of distress, it healed my mind and heart of past hurt and pain, and, when I thought there was no way out, it taught me that all things are possible with God. When I could not be satisfied by anything in life, the Word filled that void and emptiness deep inside. When I was agitated, stressed, and depressed, the Word of God calmed my body, relaxed my mind, and put my spirit at rest. The bottom line is, there is power in the Word of God. There is the power to change your mind, your heart, your whole being, and the power to transform your life. Hebrews 4:12 reads, *"For the word of God is living and powerful, and sharper than any two-edged sword, piercing even to the division of soul and spirit, and of joints and marrow, and is a discerner of the thoughts and intents of the heart."*

The Word can help you learn how to overcome life's challenges, teach you how to walk in victory, and how to have joy and peace in your life regardless of your circumstances. It is the preacher's and Bible teacher's job or duty to make the Word relevant so that you can apply it to your life.

But some are not preaching the Word. They misrepresent the character of God and the power of God by "pimping the people." They say what they think will tickle the ear rather than what will help people overcome their problems. I have seen it over and over in ministry, and I pray to God that it will stop. Paul addresses false prophets and false teachers throughout his writings. He tells us to beware of them.

So read the Bible for yourself! If you don't read it for yourself, how do you know that what you hear in church is actually coming from the mouth of God or whether it's the preacher's opinions or thoughts? Whenever I hear the word being preached, I decipher what comes from God and what comes from man, and if I'm not sure I look it up for myself. I don't accept everything that is said just because a "man or woman of God" said it. I want to hear what God has to say because that is the only thing that delivered my soul and put my mind at rest.

Pray to God

In addition to reading the Bible, prayer is necessary to find spiritual rest and develop a personal relationship with God. However, prayer seems to be very difficult for many Christians. I believe one of the reasons prayer is so difficult is that it's not natural to talk to someone you cannot see, hear, or touch in the way we do with other human beings. Some people tell me they feel strange speaking into the air when they are supposed to be talking to God. I believe other people have trouble praying because, for the most part, it doesn't provide immediate results. We're a quick-fix society and many of us do not have patience. We want fast food, fast weight loss, and a fast answer to our prayers.

It also seems to me that men have a harder time praying than women. It may be because men believe in being physical and prayer appears inactive. Also, men in our society are seen as authority figures, so praying could seem like admitting a need for help or being inferior to a superior God.

Many Christians pray openly during church services or meetings, but find it hard to spend personal time praying to God regularly. Even some church leaders, ministers, preachers, and teachers of the Word of God are so busy working for God they don't have time to pray to God.

Being a Christian means to have the characteristics of Christ. Jesus lived a life of prayer. He often withdrew from the crowd to seek the Father's presence for spiritual renewal and strength. He also went to his Father in prayer for guidance and direction.

Can you imagine working for a company where you are so busy you never have time to find out your next work assignment? That is what it's like living without praying, meditating, and listening to what God wants you to do. You may wear yourself out doing something, only to find out that this was not your assignment.

Prayer is essential for spiritual rest. Prayer is a way to control your hunger pangs for God. It is necessary in order to find that inner peace, in order to lie beside the still waters; to help you lie down in the green pasture of God so that you may have rest in your inner man. And this rest in your inner world will help you better handle the stress and challenges of your physical world.

What exactly is prayer? I have heard many descriptions. Some say it's intimacy with God, communing with God, talking to God, spending quality time with God, acknowledging God, thanking God, making requests of God, getting strength and guidance from God, worshiping and praising God, confessing faults and acknowledging the need for help from God, or just communication with God. Prayer includes all of these descriptions.

Let's go straight to the Word to see what the Word (John 1:1) has to say about prayer.

In Luke 18:1–8, Jesus tells a parable to illustrate the need for constant prayer. It's a parable about a persistent woman. He begins in verse 1 by saying *"that men always ought to pray and not lose heart."* Then He continues with the parable. You can read it in detail for yourself. But to sum it up, a judge granted this woman's request because she persistently came to the judge seeking justice. Jesus says that if an unjust judge can give this woman her request because of her constantly coming to him, won't God, who is the God of justice, answer His people who also constantly come to him? I can especially relate to this as a parent. Sometimes just the mere persistence of my children may get them their requests.

He wants us to come to Him persistently, not begging, but keeping our requests before Him (Philippians 4:4) and believing He will answer our prayers.

God promises to answer us, He just doesn't tell us when. The answer may not come on our time schedule, but God does answer prayers. So when you pray, don't get discouraged if the answer or result doesn't come when you want it to. Be persistent like the persistent woman, and believe by faith that God will answer your prayers. Jeremiah 33:3 reads, *"Call to Me and I will answer you, and show you great and mighty things, which you did not know."*

I really love the next illustration Jesus uses in Luke 18:10–14. I have spoken to many people who think they are not worthy to pray to God or are ashamed because they feel they are not as committed to God as they should be. Other people tell me they don't know how to pray because they don't use all of the theological words or may not be fluent or knowledgeable in biblical studies. However, in this particular parable Jesus resolves this issue. He tells a story of two men who went to pray in the temple. One was a Pharisee, who belonged to a sect of religious people who lived by the law. The other man was a tax collector. The Pharisee very pridefully and arrogantly prayed to God, telling God how righteous he was and how he wasn't like other sinners or the tax collector. The tax collector also prayed to God, but humbled himself before the Lord and admitted his faults. The tax collector returned home forgiven by God; the Pharisee did not.

This illustration demonstrates what I love so much about praying to God. No matter where you are in your life, you can come to God just as you are. Just speak to Him. You don't have to use certain biblical terms, be a student of theological studies, or be eloquent in speech. God knows everything about each of us anyway, so we can be completely open and honest with Him about anything and everything in our lives.

That doesn't mean that we come to God disrespectfully. We should revere God and come with a humble heart before the Almighty God, the Creator of the universe. But you don't have to try to impress God. And you sure don't have to be perfect to pray to God. As a matter of fact, there are no perfect people. The Bible says, "... *for all have sinned and fallen short of the glory of God ...*" (Romans 3:23). The Pharisee's problem was that he came to God as though he were perfect instead of acknowledging his faults. He was wrong to think he was better than others and to put them down rather than help them.

Praise God. Through Jesus Christ we can come boldly before the throne that we may obtain mercy and find grace to help us in time of need (Hebrews 4:16). You can let your hair down and take off the mask you may have been wearing throughout the day. You can be real with God because He knows exactly where you are in your life and who you really are. The Bible says He even knows what you need before you ask Him.

I used to think if God knew everything, then why did I need to ask Him for anything? However, prayer is more than just asking God to meet your needs as if He is Santa Claus, a "sugar daddy," or the "candy man." God created us to have fellowship with Him. God wants us to know Him intimately, and prayer will help us establish a personal relationship with a personal God. Prayer will help satisfy that part of us that yearns to be connected with our Maker instead of trying to fill the void with physical desires such as food, alcohol, drugs, sex, money, or power.

Often when I had the desire to overeat, I went to God in prayer and just screamed out, "Lord, I need help!"

Just like David said he cried out to the Lord and the Lord delivered him, the Lord helped me, but I also had to learn how to listen to God for instructions. That's when I realized that prayer is not just talking to God, but talking *with* God. Prayer isn't just asking God for what you want, but also asking Him what *He* wants for you. He created every human being with a specific purpose in mind. When you pray, don't just get in the habit of asking for your desires. Ask God to line up your life with *His* will so you can be all that He created you to be.

I used to think I had an excellent prayer life because I talked to God all day, every day. Whether I was working, shopping, exercising, or doing chores in the house, I spoke out loud or talked to Him quietly. But one day I finally realized I was not truly communicating with God, because communication is also listening. I couldn't just keep asking God for help. I had to learn what He wanted me to do for this temple He created. I could not control my problem, but He could. I had to learn how to listen to God so He could direct my steps and tell me how to control my mouth. When you pray, don't just present your requests before God, but learn how to listen.

You may be wondering if you will hear an audible voice come down from heaven with lightning bolts and thunder. Sorry, but that is not how it happens. Remember, God spoke to Elijah with a small, quiet voice. Many of us don't ever get to hear that small, still voice of God because we're too busy doing all of the talking or we are not still or quiet enough to hear it. Some people pray, then immediately stop praying after they've expressed their needs or wants.

I have been guilty of this myself on many occasions. I have talked *at* God rather than *with* God. God could be ready to give a clear answer, but we sometimes jump up too quickly or stop listening too soon.

Prayer is also a great way to begin and end each day. Even if you go through your daily activities in a prayerful mind, it is important to set aside a specific time to pray so that you can have personal fellowship with God. Prayer first thing in the morning can get you off to a great start, as King David said in Psalm 63. And prayer at night can put your spirit at rest to help you have a peaceful sleep. In Matthew 6:6, Jesus said, *"But you, when you pray, go into your room, and when you have shut your door, pray to your Father who is in the secret place; and your Father who sees in secret will reward you openly."*

Have a secret place and a specific time just for you and God to spend quality time. The more time you spend with Him, the more you will get to know His voice. But how will you ever hear the voice of God speaking to your heart if you don't take the time to listen? How will you know the answers He is trying to give you to specific questions if you don't take the time to recognize His voice? How will you know His will for your life, or what is right for your body, His temple, if you don't listen to His plans for you, including your eating and exercise habits? Do what Samuel did when he was ready to hear from God in I Samuel, Chapter 3. Samuel said, *"Speak Lord for Your servant hears."* Then the Lord spoke to Samuel.

You may feel like some people who say they don't know how to pray. There are different prayer postures. The one that Christians are more familiar with is praying while kneeling, palms together in front of the face. However, in biblical times people prayed prostrate, face and stomach down with their bodies stretched out on the ground, or standing while bowing their heads. There is actually no single correct posture; it is just important to come with a humble spirit.

Although Marcus, my client, began to change by reading the Word, he found prayer extremely difficult.

Marcus found kneeling difficult and said it felt strange to pray to someone he couldn't see and who did not immediately respond to him. He and his wife started praying together, but she did all of the talking and he did all of the listening to her prayers. So I suggested that he write to God. This was very effective for him and eventually he felt more comfortable praying in the standard posture, talking to God. When he wrote in his journal he did fine, but when he started speaking, he did not know what to say to God. Jesus resolved this in Matthew 6:9–13 and in Luke 11:2–4 when His disciples asked Him to teach them how to pray. He taught them what is commonly referred to as the Lord's Prayer.

Our Father in heaven,
Hallowed be Your name.
Your kingdom come.
Your will be done
On earth as it is in heaven.
Give us this day our daily bread.
And forgive us our debts,
As we forgive our debtors.
And do not lead us into temptation,
But deliver us from the evil one.
For Yours is the kingdom and the power and the glory forever.
Amen.

Jesus gives us a model for praying. If you do pray this prayer, don't just memorize it and quote it out of habit. Read it and think about what it means so that it won't be meaningless and come from your mouth from memory only and not from your heart. It shows how we should give praise and honor to a holy God, who is also our loving

Father; how we need to pray for His will to be done not only in our lives but on the earth; how we can rely on God to supply us with our daily needs; how we need to ask for forgiveness as we also are to forgive others; and how we can ask Him to help us in our times of trials and temptations from the devil. Even when you speak to God in your own words, think about this pattern and begin with praising and thanking God for who He is, pray for the world and His will to be done, pray for God to meet your needs, pray for forgiveness and for others, and pray that He helps you in times of trouble. Instead of relying on external stimuli to satisfy that inner unrest and hunger, pray to your heavenly Father and allow Him to provide the peace and assurance for your restless soul.

Study Scripture

MATTHEW 11:28–30

Come to Me, all you who labor and are heavy laden, and I will give you rest. Take My yoke upon you and learn from Me, for I am gentle and lowly in heart, and you will find rest for your souls. For My yoke is easy and my burden is light.

PRAYER

Dear God,
Thank you for loving me so much that you gave me the gift of life through your precious Spirit. I now know that I am fearfully and wonderfully made and marvelous are Your works, as the Scriptures say (Psalms 139:14). I want to care for my body, the temple of God, so I can be the best you created me to be. Fill my inner longings with the presence of your Spirit. Satisfy my cravings with the flavor of your Word. Heal my broken spirit through the power of prayer. Help me commit to reading your word and spending quality time alone with you. Forgive me for being so

concerned about the cares of this world that I have neglected the most essential things necessary for the survival of my soul. Early will I seek you in prayer because I now know that my flesh is longing for the living God alone. I cast all of my cares on you and I will not worry about tomorrow. I will meditate on your goodness as you teach me how to take one day at a time, step by step. I am relying on Your strength, on Your promises, and on Your presence to calm my spirit and put to rest my longing soul. In Jesus' name I pray. Amen.

ACTIVITIES

1. Record your Study Scriptures on index cards. I used a spiral index-card holder to carry my cards with me in my purse. I read and studied first thing in the morning before I started my day at work, for at least five minutes during my lunchtime, and at night before I went to bed. Find the times that work for you. Carrying them with me was extremely helpful when I got the desire to over-eat. So when you get those outrageous urges and you know you will overeat, feast on God's Word instead.

Here is a list of some of the many Scriptures that helped me gain control over my appetite and encouraged me to care for my body by eating healthier and having the desire to exercise:

Joshua 1:8–9
Psalms 23:1; 107:20
Proverbs 3:5–6; 12:1; 13:25
Matthew 4:4; 5:6; 6:33; 11:28–30
Acts 1:8
Ephesians 3:20; 6:10
I Thessalonians 5:23
I Peter 2:9

Jude vv. 24–25
Revelation 3:8–13, 20; 12:11

2. Evaluate your sleeping pattern for one week. During this time answer the following questions: Is your sleep consistent? (Do you go to bed at approximately the same time each day?) Do you get quality sleep? Do you wake up refreshed and renewed or do you struggle to wake up each morning? How do you think you can improve your sleep?

3. Make a list of—and reflect on—your positive lifestyle changes. Also write down at least three other areas in which you would like to improve, and include a plan for improvement.

4. Pray each and every time before you eat, asking God to direct your eating during that meal or snack time. Also begin and end your day with prayer. Practice this until it becomes a natural part of your life. If you ever had uncontrollable desires to overeat like I did, there may be times when reading or meditating on your Scriptures is not enough. In some instances, you may find it hard to concentrate, depending on what the stressor is. In this case pray, pray, pray. Call out to God so he can strengthen you and help you. Before you know it, your mind will be off the food as you begin to enjoy this special time with God.

5. Choose one day of the week that you practice spending quiet time with God. Begin by reading a Scripture. Now take deep, slow breaths. Meditate on the Scripture. Slowly, move into prayer. Begin by thanking God, then spend quiet time listening. You don't have to limit this activity to one day a week. As a matter of fact, when you see how peaceful and relaxing it is to commune with the Almighty Creator, you will realize you need to do it more often.

6. Try to boost up your exercise routine and energy expenditure. If you have been walking, walk more briskly with longer strides, swinging your arms faster. You can walk with small dumbbells in your hands to add an upper body resistance workout as well. Or you can combine walking with short bouts of jogging. If you have been jogging, try doing some short bursts of sprints or choose a path with more hills. Add some stair climbing to your routine. If you're doing aerobics, consciously increase your intensity level with each movement or try a more advanced class if you're ready for it. Whatever you do, consciously increase your intensity level. Listen to your body, don't overexert yourself, and enjoy spicing up your workout.

Get rid of the excuses that stop you from being "fit for God"

1. Pursuit of Money

We all need money to pay our bills and live a comfortable life, but what is the purpose in constantly working to make more money if it causes sorrow and poor health or if you won't be around long enough to enjoy it? Health is wealth. **I Timothy 6:10** *For the love of money is the root of all kinds of evil, for which some have strayed from the faith in their greediness, and pierced themselves through with many sorrows.*

2. Lack of Peace

Jesus told His disciples that He was leaving them His peace. His peace is the peace that the world cannot understand. It will have you laughing instead of crying, singing instead of screaming, and praising God instead of throwing in the towel. But you have to take hold of it by trusting in the Prince of Peace. **Isaiah 26:3** *You will keep him in perfect peace, whose mind is stayed on You, because he trusts in You.*

3. Impatience

Don't give up when you don't see results as fast as you would like. And don't compare yourself to others. If you keep doing what it takes, your results will be well worth the wait. **Psalm 37:7–9** *Rest in the Lord, and wait patiently for Him; do not fret because of him who* *prospers in his way, because of the man who brings wicked schemes to pass. Cease from anger, and forsake wrath; do not fret—it only causes harms. For evildoers shall be cut off; but those who wait on the Lord, they shall inherit the earth.*

4. FATIGUE

See a doctor to make sure you don't have a medical condition and make sure you get sufficient rest. Physical fatigue can be a manifestation of mental fatigue, which can also make you feel sluggish and drained. Pray and ask God to help you and rely on His strength to get you through the day. **Isaiah 41:10** *Fear not, for I am with you; Be not dismayed, for I am your God. I will strengthen you, yes, I will help you, I will uphold you with My righteous right hand.*

5. GRIEF

Grief is a normal part of human life. Although we may never stop missing our loved ones, the loss will get easier to bear in time. God is the giver of life and the author of death, so we can have comfort in trusting our loved ones in His care. **II Corinthians 5:8** *We are confident, yes, well pleased rather to be absent from the body and to be present with the Lord.*

Week Eight
Share and Be Prepared

Then God Blessed Them, and God Said to Them, Be
Fruitful and Multiply . . .
—Genesis 1:28

The story of creation demonstrates how God brought a vast universe into being by speaking it into existence. It also shows how important humankind is to God, more important than any other creation. God prepared and shaped the earth specifically to accommodate man's existence. Then He made humankind in His own image and gave him dominion over the earth. After God prepared the earth and created man, He gave him two basic commands that I am going to discuss during Week Eight to help you maintain your results and be prepared for the battles ahead.

The first command is in Genesis 1:28 when the Lord blessed Adam and Eve and told them to "be fruitful and to multiply." The Lord was telling Adam and Eve to have children and increase in number. I like the word "fruitful." What distinguishes a fruit is the fact that it has seed within itself to produce more fruit like itself that can produce more fruit, and so on.

But how can this be relevant to weight management? One of the most important things you can do is to "be fruitful." As you go through each week, as you learn how to live healthier, as you put new tips into practice, don't keep it all to yourself. Share with others. Start planting positive seeds of success in other lives until finally you have multiplied.

I believe success in any area of life is not determined by the status you have achieved, by your degree, your neighborhood, who you know, the car you drive, or how much money you make. I believe true success is sharing with others what you have learned and achieved. In doing this you're not trying to make little "images of yourself." How boring the world would be if we were all alike. Instead, you want to share the qualities and principles that give birth to success.

Jesus Christ Himself mentions the importance of bearing "fruit" throughout the New Testament. In John 15:8, He says, *"By this My Father is glorified, that you bear much fruit; so you will be My disciples."* And in John 15:16, He sums up His whole reason for choosing His followers: *"You did not choose Me, but I chose you and appointed you that you should go and bear fruit, and that your fruit should remain . . ."*

This was the main reason Jesus chose twelve disciples who walked with Him and witnessed His many miracles, His life, His death, and His resurrection. He was preparing them to be sent out to spread the message of salvation throughout Israel as preparation for the worldwide mission to follow. He chose them so that after His death they could preach about Him as eyewitnesses. Having a firsthand account and knowledge of his ministry, they could share their witness with others. Jesus wanted them to "bear much fruit" by making more disciples. This was their ultimate mission and purpose. In Matthew 28:19, Jesus gave His disciples the "great commission" when he said, *"Go therefore and make disciples of all the nations, baptizing them in the name of the Father and of the Son and of the Holy Spirit . . ."*

Jesus' disciples were people of various backgrounds, careers, races, and differences. But they had the same common goal of striving to be successful in this life by obtaining eternal life and of sharing the good news of Christ. Just as Christ tells the importance of bearing fruit, He also mentions that if a tree does not bear fruit it will be destroyed, like the fig tree that withered because it did not bear any fruit. Look at this Scripture in Luke 13:9, *"And if it bears fruit well. But if not, after that you can cut it down."*

I believe that this biblical concept can also apply to weight management. It's amazing how sharing your success with others can actually benefit you, while keeping it to yourself can work against you down the road. Sharing with others helps you keep and maintain an attitude of wellness because you create a network of people who will lift you up when you need encouragement. When we don't share, we stay focused on our own issues and our own struggles, which can make change more difficult.

Galatians 6:7 reads, *"Do not be deceived, God is not mocked; for whatever a man sows, that he will also reap."* As you plant good seeds into your own life, seeds of healthier eating, seeds of caring for your body, seeds of exercising, and seeds of having a positive attitude, share with others and your harvest is sure to come. Galatians 6:9 says, *"And let us not grow weary while doing good, for in due season we shall reap if we do not lose heart."* According to the Word of God, which is the truth of God, if you keep doing what you need to do—don't give up but wait for it—you will get the results you want.

Use the creativity He's given you and apply this great biblical principle. Plant seeds of success in your life and other people's lives. Reach out and bear an abundance of fruit by sharing with others. In I Timothy 6:17 it states that it is God who gives us richly all things to enjoy. Verse 18 speaks on the importance of sharing with others. Although in this particular passage earthly riches are mentioned, this principle applies to all good things God has made available to us.

Here are some examples of how you can share with others in order to start bearing fruit.

1. Greet someone. Speak to people to whom you don't normally speak. It has always amazed me how two of God's greatest creations can walk right past one another and not even acknowledge each other. Even dogs acknowledge each other's presence with a bark, a wag of the tail, a sniff, or a growl. When you see someone walking around the track, say hello. Speak to others in your exercise class. Speak to your neighbor. Do you even know who your neighbors are? When you go in the grocery store, speak to the grocery clerks. Say thank you and show your appreciation for their service. It's amazing how a "How are you doing?" or a simple smile can go a long way to brighten someone else's day.

2. Don't entertain negativity. I believe attitudes are contagious. Negative people exert negative energy: being positive creates positive energy. I've been around a lot of people who really didn't have anything good to say about anyone or anything, and I have learned to do two things in this situation: (a) I don't contribute to their negativity, and (b) I try to acknowledge the positive in the situation. For Christ said that we are to be the light of the world and, *"Let your light shine before men, that they may see your good works and glorify your Father in heaven"* (Matthew 5:16). Because I stayed focused on the positive and did not contribute to their negative comments, these people quickly learned they can't bring negativity to me. Some of them eventually changed their attitudes, or perhaps they just changed them around me.

Negativity includes complaining, gossiping, backbiting, criticizing, and degrading others. If you participate, you're planting negativity in your own spirit, which hinders your progress toward healthier living. Sprinkle positive seeds over those negative weeds and watch your fruit grow.

3. Buy bottled water and share. You don't have to do this often, but try it and see what happens. I bought bottled water and placed it on my coworkers' desks to encourage them and remind them of the importance of drinking water. For many people it worked. They started bringing in their own bottled water to keep at their desks for convenience. I was also blessed because many of them gave me water and shared information, telling me where and when the cases were on sale. Keeping bottles of water at home encouraged my children to drink more water. They found it more convenient to grab a bottle of water than to pour a glass from the refrigerator.

4. Make a fruit basket. Instead of baking cakes, pies, or cookies to give away, make a fruit basket to encourage healthy eating. Include a variety of colorful fruits, a box of raisins, a healthy trail mix, and a small book, like a promise book or a miniature Bible. Be creative and discover ways of sharing the gift of health with someone else.

5. Make a plant dish. Plants are definitely a demonstration of the life-giving ability and power of God. I love to start them as young plants and watch them grow. I also take clippings off of my mature plants and start new plants to share with others. Purchase a plant to give to someone or repot one of your starter plants. Buy a vase and colorful rocks, fill the vase with water, put in clippings, and give it as a gift. Most people appreciate the beauty of plants, whether they have a "green thumb" or not.

6. Support a marathon or walk. Many marathons and walks are held now to support research and cures for all kinds of illnesses. Many of these groups also provide training for you. Even if you decide not to physically participate, you can cheer on others, help raise money, or support them by being a sponsor or giving a donation. Reach out and show someone that you care.

7. Start an exercise group. You don't have to be a fitness guru to start an exercise class. If space is available where you work, contact a local fitness center to see if instructors are available to come in and teach. Many different types of classes are available where you don't have to jump around and sweat until you drop, which can be a deterrent for exercising on the job.

Another idea is to invite a fitness trainer, nutritionist, or other health expert to come and speak during a lunch hour about the benefits of healthier living. Organize a walking group to share the gift of fitness with others. Walk around the block or up and down the stairs at lunch, during breaks, or before or after work.

8. Send someone a card with words of encouragement. Every person knows someone who is going through a difficult time. Even if you don't know what to say or how to encourage someone who may be experiencing grief or a difficult situation, send a card of support and reassurance to show that you care. Remember, fitness starts from the inside out, and when someone is going through a traumatic experience, the last thing they may think about is eating right or eating at all—and they don't really feel like exercising. But knowing that someone else cares could be the special boost a person needs to stay uplifted and motivated until the storm subsides.

9. E-mail a prayer, Scripture, or health tips. Many people now spend hours each day on their computer either at home or on the job. E-mailing a Scripture, prayer, or health tip can be a refreshing break after spending so much time engrossed in work. E-mailing is a great way to give someone a lift.

Send a message to a group of friends, family members, or coworkers and ask them to send it to others with a note that they share it also. Before you know it, your message has blessed more people than you ever imagined.

10. Share with the forgotten. Thousands of people in our society seem to have been forgotten—the sick, the handicapped, the elderly, and others. They are God's beautiful creations, just as we are. But many people don't want to deal with the reality of aging or of being sick or physically disabled. I used to wonder why I didn't see many elderly or disabled people in my everyday life. Then I learned, I had to go to them. Volunteer at a nursing home or hospital, visit someone and share words of encouragement, or read to a sick child.

Most of us wouldn't struggle so much with our own issues if we reached out and shared the precious gift of love and care with others. When you reach out to others, your problems don't seem so big.

Although not all of the tips are about eating or exercising, they all have a direct impact on being physically healthy. Fitness starts from the inside out. If you begin sharing positive experiences with others, not only will you feel better on the inside so you can take better care of your outside, you will also contribute to the positive attitude and welfare of others. I mentioned earlier that attitudes are contagious. Plant good seeds and watch the harvest grow. Be fruitful and multiply.

Adam and Eve were in the beautiful garden God created and prepared especially for them. They could pick fresh fruit off of the beautiful fruit trees; they could walk beside the flowing rivers of water and lie down for a refreshing nap in the beautiful green grass. God told them to be fruitful and multiply, and God gave them everything they could ever need for success. But one day they had to face temptation, and their world as they knew it changed.

As you are learning how to live healthier and you begin to share with others, be aware that temptation will come. What you have obtained, learned, and shared with others will be put to the test.

In Genesis 2:16, the Lord commanded man to freely eat of every tree of the garden, except from the tree of the knowledge of good and evil. He told him that the day he ate of that tree, he would die. In Genesis, Chapter 3, the serpent, an extremely cunning beast of the field, deceived the woman and got her to doubt what God said.

Adam and Eve had everything they needed. God personally came to them right in the garden, yet temptation came also and they ate the forbidden fruit.

I have my own testimony about sharing with others and being challenged by temptation. I had gone through so much with weight loss and overeating, and finally I was on the right track. I lost the weight, overcame depression, stopped bingeing, and was growing in the knowledge of God. I was very active in ministry and was teaching classes, workshops, and seminars at churches, retreats, conferences, and health fairs around the country. I had been on TBN and *The 700 Club,* and I was producing my own fitness television show and videos. God had truly blessed me and delivered me, so I just wanted to help everybody I could. Then finally it seemed like a flood of tests came one after the other.

After I had surgery on both knees, it seemed as time passed I was experiencing more and more stiffness. I couldn't walk up stairs without holding on to the side rail for support. The colder and wetter it was outside, the more stiffness and pain I felt. I had to limit my days of aerobic activity to avoid living with constant knee pain. Then I was in a car accident. I was sitting at a light waiting for it to turn green when a tractor-trailer slammed right into the back of my car. I asked God: How can I continue to be a fitness instructor and help others live healthier if the very tool I need to do this is being broken down?

I began to question the vision God had given me about a fitness ministry, my fitness television program, videos, and even this book. Things seemed to get worse in every way. The pastor I had loved and respected for years got sick and died. Then I became a member of another ministry, and to my surprise and shock there were strong rumors of sexual immorality among the leadership and of large amounts of money missing.

During this time I also met and married my husband, Roberto. And although marriage is a beautiful experience, it was also another new challenge to my life. I met Roberto at one of the fitness centers where I taught aerobics classes and was a personal trainer. When I met him, he expressed his desire to lose weight and learn how to eat healthier. He ate fast food almost every day, snacked frequently, drank sodas, and seldom drank water. Just as I had done in the past, he used food as a comfort and as his drug of choice. I thought I could help him overcome his challenges because I had helped so many other people. But I soon found out that this challenge was emotionally draining because the client was someone so close to me.

Roberto needed healing from his past and healing from the grief of losing his mother. He was on an emotional roller-coaster ride that manifested itself in bouts of overeating, depression, and anger. He bought snacks and kept them in the house for munching. In the beginning it didn't bother me at all and I didn't feel tempted. But as I was exposed to more and more of his negativity, I felt more and more tempted to grab something to eat. Surrounded by more negativity than I'd experienced in years, I started buying more snacks.

In the beginning of this book I mentioned the importance of staying focused on the positive and finding the good in negative situations. Believe me; I was truly put to the test. Roberto is an intelligent, college-educated, hardworking man, but I also began to think of him as a person who had a gift for finding the negative in the positive. I don't care how great the news was; he found the potential problem in it. In retrospect I believe this attitude was most likely caused by the many disappointments in his life. He expected the worst to happen so he wouldn't be disappointed if something went wrong. It was his way of protecting his emotions from further harm.

Like most people who want to lose weight, he was very impatient. When he didn't see results fast enough, he gave up. In the meantime, I found myself overindulging in food with or without him. I wholeheartedly wanted to help him, but the more I tried, the more I somehow found myself slipping backward and eating more high-calorie, fattening foods and snacking. I had overcome many issues from my past, but now new experiences, new emotions, and a lot of frustration caused me to crave snacks again. I took a seat on Roberto's emotional roller-coaster ride and on many days found myself totally out of control. I ate when I wasn't hungry or when I knew

I shouldn't be eating. I remember running out to the grocery store to buy a pint of Häagen-Dazs butter pecan ice cream, a box of microwave butter popcorn, Mrs. Fields chocolate chip cookies, and a container of Tums for indigestion.

I used food to relax, to reward myself, to celebrate working hard all week, or for accomplishing another goal in life. Food became my comfort and my friend again. For the first time in almost ten years I began to lose what I had worked so hard to gain.

The rolls and cellulite were back on my thighs, I lost my small waistline, my stomach began to bulge out, and I didn't feel energetic. When I exercised I immediately got tired. And after my bouts of overeating I had a hangover that left me lethargic and most times without the energy or motivation to exercise. In less than two years I gained over twenty pounds and had to buy a completely new wardrobe.

This vicious cycle snuck in slowly. I don't remember gaining the first five or ten pounds. I was so busy focusing on Roberto and his issues that I didn't realize I was slipping.

In this way I learned some very valuable lessons about trying to help others. First of all, you cannot try to help others at your own expense, no matter who they are. I learned that I was not equipped to be God in anyone's life. That is why God sent his Son, Jesus Christ, to die on the cross for the world. He's the Savior; I'm just a messenger.

People need to make the decision to deal with their issues and live healthier for themselves. It's a personal choice. Even God Himself gives us a choice. We weren't created to be robots, but to have a free will to make decisions. Deuteronomy 30:1 reads, "... I have set before you life and death, blessing and cursing; therefore choose life, that both you and your descendants may live . . ." This verse tells us that our choices can also affect our family members or loved ones. For example, children can learn poor eating habits from their parents and then later teach their own children. But God says you have a choice, choose life.

In John, Chapter 5, there's a story about a pool in Jerusalem that was called Bethesda and had five porches. On these porches lay a great multitude of sick people, blind, lame, and paralyzed. They lay there waiting for the water to move, for at a certain time an angel would come down and stir up the water and whoever stepped in first, after the stirring of the water, was made well of whatever disease he had. A man was lying there who had been sick for thirty-eight long years. When Jesus saw him lying there, He said to him, "Do you want to be made well?" The sick man answered that whenever the water was stirred, he had no one to put him in the pool. Jesus' response was, *"Rise, take up your bed and walk."* After thirty-eight long years, the man's problem had become a way of life for him. What Jesus was telling him was that if he wanted things to change, he had to get up and do something about it.

The truth is, some people don't really want to change for various reasons, although they may complain about their situation. This man probably made his living from begging and had become comfortable receiving sympathy from others. Once healed, he was going to have to get up and be accountable for his life.

As you and I are going along and sharing with others, we need to be aware that there will be people you may desperately want to share with or help, but each person may not wholeheartedly want his life to change. Change involves taking responsibility for one's own actions. As I was working with Roberto, I noticed that he often spoke of wanting things to change, but when it was time to really do something about it, he always had an excuse. And whenever he got upset or angry it was always because of what somebody else did to him. His focus for blame was always on others and never on himself.

I can definitely relate to him feeling this way because in my past

I always blamed my situation on other people. I said I overate because of my childhood, or because my father was an alcoholic, or because I was a single parent, one excuse after the other. But the change couldn't take place in my body until I made a decision in my mind that I truly wanted things to change. It wasn't my husband who made me overeat and neglect my body. I chose to allow stress and frustration to take control of me. I learned that neither your condition, your experiences, nor your past has to dictate your future. It's up to you to get up and do something about it.

Hebrews 12:1–2 reads, *"Therefore we also, since we are surrounded by so great a cloud of witnesses, let us lay aside every weight, and the sin which so easily ensnares us, and let us run with endurance the race that is set before us, looking unto Jesus, the author and finisher of our faith . . ."* This Scripture tells us that we are to lay aside anything that prevents us from wholeheartedly living our lives to the fullness that God intends for us. God doesn't want us to allow our circumstances to weigh us down and endanger our physical and spiritual health. I felt myself burdened down with Roberto's weight and my new weight gain. I no longer had the energy and stamina I once had, but I realized I had to let go and keep my eyes focused on Christ so that I could hold on to what I had worked so hard to gain. I made the choice that I would continue to strive for health and would not give up.

So always be willing to share with others, but remember that it is up to them to make the decision to change. By sharing information you plant seeds that can grow at the appropriate time, which is God's time. Sharing with others can definitely help keep you motivated, but do not help them by risking your own health. Know when your job is done and then pray and trust God for the rest. And yes, it is harder when these people you try to share with are your loved ones or friends, but that is when you truly have to have faith in God. Remember that the same God that was there to help you can help them also.

As I was going through my challenge with my health, the church, and my husband, the devil cunningly got me to question what God had said. Satan used my desire to help others against me, and he tempted me in a way in which I had not been tempted in years. It was just like the way he got Eve to doubt God and pick the fruit.

The extra weight not only made me feel less energetic and affected my clothes size and appearance, but it also made me have PMS symptoms like I have never experienced before. When I told my doctor that my PMS symptoms were getting increasingly worse, she told me that weight gain and becoming less active could definitely play a major role in these new symptoms. Neglecting my health added to PMS—a "perfect moment for Satan."

I knew I had to lose weight. I wanted to feel better and look better again. I made up my mind that I was going to get up and do something about it. I was determined that food and being around negativity were not going to have control over me anymore. Just as God called light into darkness, I was going to make some new changes in my life. However, as I began to focus on the positive, my greatest temptation was no longer the food; it was how to get off the weight. I was no longer in the same body I had years ago when I first lost weight. I was now limited in my aerobic and exercise capacity, and I was almost forty years old. Believe me, losing over twenty pounds in an almost forty-year-old body seemed much harder than losing over fifty pounds in a twenty-five-year-old body. My energy level and enthusiasm just were not the same.

Also nowadays we're seeing so many new diets out there. Even on my job everybody was involved in some type of diet program, and I actually saw many people lose weight. I was tempted to try one of these programs because I wanted the weight off so badly. After everything I'd gone through in my past trying to lose weight the right way, now temptation was staring me right in the face every day. In my home I faced snacks, at church it was the temptation to overeat those fattening dinners, and on my job I wrestled with my desire to try a quick-fix diet.

I went to the weight loss section in the grocery and drug stores and read the labels on all of the new products available. I actually put some diet items in my cart and walked around the store for at least thirty minutes before I put them back on the shelf. The diet industry sent messages to me everywhere I went. I pondered buying the new fat-burning products, the new shakes, drinks, and pills and books on protein diets, low-carb diets, and grapefruit diets. Then to make the temptation hotter, all I saw on the fronts of magazines in the food checkout lines was "Lose 20 pounds," "Lose 30 pounds," or "How I lost 50 pounds." I flipped through magazines that had beautiful bodies on the covers and read one story after another on dieting.

The people on my job weighed themselves every day and lost weight fast on many of the quick-fix diets. But I saw many of them immediately gain back the weight and struggle week after week, which reminded me of the failure in quick fixes. It had been so long that I had forgotten how desperate you feel when you want the weight off. So what do you do when these trials and temptations come your way?

I wish I could end this book by telling you that once you have lost weight all of your cares and worries are over. But that's not the truth or the reality of life. Just as the Bible tells us to work out our own salvation, living healthy is something you will have to work out daily. Even if you heal from what is troubling you from your past or lock the trigger that makes you overeat, there will always be a new trial or temptation in your life. And that doesn't mean you are doing anything wrong. Whether you're a minister, a choir member, an usher at the door, the pastor, the president of the United States, a CEO of a multimillion-dollar company, a secretary, or a housewife, you will experience the trials and temptations of life at one time or another.

Jesus Christ said, *"In the world you will have tribulation; but be of good cheer, I have overcome the world"* (John 16:33).

The great biblical characters faced various trials. Shadrach, Meshach, and Abed-nego were thrown into a fiery furnace because they would not bow down and serve a false god; Daniel was thrown in a lion's den because others were jealous of him; Joseph was sold into slavery by his own brothers, then forgotten in prison after being falsely accused of a crime. And we all have heard about the story of Job and how he lost everything he had and was accused of sinning by his friends because of his tragedy. But the Bible says he was a righteous man.

The Bible is full of many more stories about the obstacles and challenges that the people of God faced. Jesus Christ himself was tempted by the devil in the wilderness. If Satan came to tempt the Son of God, of course he's going to tempt you and me. But we can overcome the temptation by following Christ's example. In Matthew, Chapter 4, He defeated the devil and overcame the temptations by knowing the Word of God. The devil tricked Eve by getting her to doubt what God had said. But if you know the Word for yourself, you can be sure of what God has said and the promises He has made available to you through His Word.

Yes, I went through new trials. Yes, I was so desperate, I was tempted to do what I knew could end in failure. But the thing that sustained me and got me back on the right track is when I read and trusted in God's word. I read how Jesus overcame temptations with the Word, I read how Shadrach, Meshach, and Abed-nego walked through the fire, and because they walked with Jesus they were not burned and did not even smell like smoke. I read how an angel of the Lord shut the mouths of the lions for Daniel and how Joseph was exalted to the highest position in the land after his trial, because he put his trust and faith in God. Job got back twice what he lost because he trusted and waited on God. And when David was mocked by his own brothers for thinking he could defeat a nine-foot-nine-inch-tall giant, he remembered his past. He looked back at what God had already done for him. He said the same God that had delivered him from the paw of the lion and bear would surely deliver him from this giant.

This is exactly how I felt when I looked back and remembered that God had delivered me in the past from overeating and from neglecting my health. He had taught me how to take care of my body before. He's the same God who had delivered me from depression, regret, and guilt. Surely He was going to be able to deliver me from this new giant and temptation in my life. He had helped me control my appetite before; He could do it again. He had created my body; therefore, He could lead me and guide me in what exercises and activities I could do in my new physical state. And as far as being in an older body, this is what Psalm 103:2–5 has to say about my health and my eating, *"Bless the Lord, O my soul, and forget not all His benefits; who forgives all your iniquities, who heals all your diseases, who redeems your life from destruction, who crowns you with loving-kindness and tender mercies, who satisfies your mouth with good things, so that your youth is renewed like the eagle's."*

So why would a good God allow His people to endure trials and temptations? Throughout the Bible trials are used to perfect us and refine us as pure gold. They are used to teach us how to rely on God's strength and his resources instead of our own. They are used to increase our faith in God. They are used to demonstrate the power of God. They are used to help create godly character in us. They are used to show us the strength we have by trusting God, and they are used so we can share with others and let them know they can be victorious in any situation. God uses trials and tests to make us better and stronger, while the devil uses temptations to try to make us fall, doubt God, and give up. But God is awesome; He can even turn the temptations of the devil around to be a tremendous blessing. For Romans 8:28 says, *"And we know that all things work together for good to those who love God, to those who are the called according to His purpose."*

When Jesus was baptized by John the Baptist in the Jordan River, God acknowledged Him as His Son in whom He was well pleased, and the Holy Spirit descended on Jesus like a dove (Matthew 3:13–17). Immediately following His baptism, Jesus was led into the wilderness by the Holy Spirit of God. After fasting for forty days and forty nights, the devil came to tempt Him. Please notice: the devil didn't come to tempt Him until He was in a weakened and vulnerable condition. Likewise, he won't try to tempt you when everything is going great and you feel absolutely wonderful. But he will come when you get some bad news, or when you have problems on your job, problems in your home, or when you're emotionally upset or in distress. Then all of a sudden you'll get this mad craving to overeat or you'll feel so down that you won't feel like exercising or even getting out of the bed. You may want to grab a cigarette or a drink to calm you down because of your nerves or stress. But remember, God allowed the devil to tempt His own Son. He knows all things, and He knew the devil would come there and tempt Jesus. Jesus was set up to be blessed, and He was. He was able to overcome each temptation with the Word of God (Matthew 4:1–11). Right after Jesus' temptation in the wilderness, His public ministry went forth powerfully with unceasing bouts of preaching, teaching, and healing. Although the devil was trying to use this wilderness experience and the temptations to try to make Christ stumble and fall, God used this experience as preparation for His public ministry. By experiencing and overcoming temptations, Jesus could now relate to others who faced various trials and temptations. He could also share by experience how to overcome them by acting on the principles found in God's Word.

This is why reading the Word of God is so important. When I read this story, God gave me an awesome revelation about my recent temptations. I realized that God still wants me to help others live healthier, but not at the expense of hurting myself or going backward. This was my true test. In the past I had overcome challenges, but many of them were from my past, so overcoming meant dealing with the mental residue or memories of the past. This time I was right in the middle of the trials and had to practice what I preached. I had to learn how to create light in the middle of darkness. Jesus said that we should be the light of the world and we should let our light shine (Matthew 5:14–16). He would not have used the word "light" if we were not going to face darkness. So I had to learn how to be successful when I faced a trial in my everyday life—in my present, not in my past.

I had already learned that God can heal you from your past, but I had to experience how it feels to still be right in the midst of the trials and temptations. Now I can tell you what I know, that you can still have peace and joy regardless of your circumstances. I can let you know from personal experience that your outside environment doesn't have to dictate how you feel on the inside. Your internal environment can change your outside.

Thank God I had a strong foundation in the Word of God that helped me endure these tests and trials. And this is why quick fixes don't work. They are temporary. When a storm or a true test comes, you'll blow right over. But by creating a strong foundation in the Word of God, you will be able to endure and eventually overcome the temptations so that you can keep what God has given you. Because of the foundation I built in God, although I got down for a moment, I didn't stay there. Proverbs 24:16 says, *"For a righteous man may fall seven times, and rise again . . ."* I knew I could get back up, experience victory in God, and share this good news with others. What the devil means for your harm, God can turn around and use as a blessing so you can be a blessing to others.

Love yourself. Love the you that God created you to be. As weird as this may sound, I am so glad I gained weight again. Although I lost a significant amount of weight in my past and overcame overeating, there was something I had missed. The way I felt about me was still based on my shape and my size. If I was small and in shape, I thought everything was okay, but when I was overweight I was not happy. I discovered that my love for myself was conditional.

Just as I had to learn how to not allow my external environment to dictate my internal peace, this time around I had to learn how to not allow my body size to dictate how I felt about myself. Although realistically, yes, I want to be in shape and look better, I must love myself with or without extra weight.

So how do you begin to love you? The Bible also says that God knew you before you were in your mother's womb. I realized that I am so special to God that He planned to give me life and thought about what He would create me to be, before I was even conceived. The Bible also says that even though we didn't even acknowledge God, didn't live for Him, and did things our own way, God still demonstrated His love for us by sending His Son, Jesus Christ, to die for all of our sins (John 3:16 and Romans 5:8). That is awesome and true love. If we could really grasp this concept of how special we are to God and how much we are loved, especially as women, we would not see all of the low self-esteem, jealousy, and envy that tear friendships apart and prevent others from happening. Looking at the stars on television and on the front covers of magazines doesn't help. I even see the jealousy, competition, and low self-esteem in the church and in ministry. If you lose weight, they say you're too small; if you gain weight, you're getting fat.

Society places so much emphasis on body size and body image that it is creating an entire population of women and teens who do not like themselves because of the unrealistic and many times "unreal" images we see. Just think about this: Although Adam and Eve had everything they ever could have wanted in the beautiful Garden of Eden, the devil was able to tempt Eve and get her to sin against God, because of what she thought she didn't have. The Bible says in Genesis 3:6, *"So when the woman saw that the tree was good for food, that it was pleasant to the eyes, and a tree desirable to make one wise, she took of its fruit and ate."*

We suffer from the same distorted beliefs today. We think if it looks good, it must be good, and we always want what we think we do not have. We also think if we look better, everything will be all right. It is true that looks may get you attention and help you make money on earth, but looks will not get you into heaven if you're ugly on the inside. Do you remember what God told the prophet Samuel when He sent him to anoint the next king of Israel? In I Samuel 16:7 the Lord told him not to look at his appearance in order to judge whether or not he was fit to be a king. Because God does not see as man sees. Man looks at the outward appearance, but God looks at the heart. I had to learn to love the person God made La Vita to be. I appreciate the gift of life that He has given me. I had to appreciate the fact that I am so special to Him and He thought so much of me that He wants the best for me. He wants me healthy and fit so I can live a more productive and fulfilling life.

This helped significantly change my focus. As long as I was focused on my body size and desperately wanting to get the weight off, I was obsessed with food and eating. But when I decided that I wanted to take better care of myself because God wanted the best for me, the obsession subsided. I was able to commit to healthy lifestyle practices while having the necessary patience to wait for the results because I wanted to be all that God had created me to be.

So don't get discouraged if you feel that you have fallen off the bandwagon or failed to lose weight. Romans 8:28 says all things work together for our good. Not only do our positive experiences help us, but our negative experiences also help us learn and grow.

Although the devil wanted to use my bad experience with a ministry to discourage me from ministry, God used it for my good.

This also meant that when my sister announced that God had placed it in her heart to pastor a church, I was open and willing to be a vessel for God's glory. I found a location for worship services and researched to find out what papers we needed to file and what licenses we needed to have. Truth, Righteousness and Love (TRL) Ministries came to fruition with my sister as the pastor and me serving as assistant to the pastor. God blessed the ministry immediately with a faithful membership and the necessary funds to get a worship location and all of the necessary work done to meet the proper building codes. The ministry is flourishing with all of the spiritual blessings of God—lives are being transformed, people are being saved, delivered, and healed, and families are being restored.

God allowed my family to be exposed to a bad ministry experience to show us that what appears bad can be turned around and used for our good. My mother is a deaconess and my older brother and younger sister are also ministers. What a blessing! It is just like my dealing with the challenge of my husband's anger and overeating. Although the experience appeared bad, I learned to stand in the midst of a fire and trust God. Roberto discovered that healing and deliverance only come from God alone. Together we discovered we had to rely on God for the answer. I learned how to have true peace and joy, which comes from the inside but can change my outside. I also learned how to put everything and everybody in the hands of God. Through my physical condition and restrictions, I learned how to rely more on God's strength and not my own.

In Joshua, Chapter 1, verses 6–9, God tells Joshua what will be the key to his success. He tells him three times in this one chapter to be strong and courageous. Joshua was now the new leader of the people of Israel, and God knew that leading people to the Promised Land would be a great and challenging task.

You and I won't have to conquer nations, but we will still face difficult situations in our everyday lives. Although there may be times when things seem tough and you won't feel like exercising, or you may be faced with other temptations, you must be strong and determined.

In Chapter 1, verse 7, God tells Joshua he must obey the rules for living found in the law of God. Likewise, if you want to be successful in weight loss, you must obey the rules. For one, if you overeat and consume more calories than you burn, you are going to gain weight. This is a simple law of energy expenditure. Extra calories in the body turn into extra fat on the body. In verse 8, God tells Joshua the importance of taking time out every day to read and meditate on the Word of God. I mentioned earlier that it was by building a strong foundation in the Word of God that I was able to get back on track and overcome temptations. However, just as God told Joshua, reading the Bible and knowing what it says is not enough. God told him to also make sure he *does* what it says. Knowing God's Word and quoting it is not enough.

Many ministers, pastors, and teachers of God's Word have preventable illnesses and diseases because they don't take care of their health. So although you may learn the Word, you have to be a doer of the Word. In James 1:22 it says that you deceive yourself when you hear the Word and don't do what it says. So just talking about wanting to live healthier, knowing what to do, and memorizing these Scriptures alone will not get you success.

After God told Joshua to meditate on the Word, He said, *"For then you will make your way prosperous, and then you will have good success."* Likewise, I have given you all of this information, but it is up to you to "make your way prosperous," or be successful in this program. It is up to you to make the commitment. There are no shortcuts to long-term results. You are going to get out of it just what you put into it. *"Whatever you sow, that you will also reap"* (Galatians 6:7).

When God gave King David's son Solomon the instructions to build a temple for God, King Solomon constructed the temple with the best supplies money could buy. He also hired the best craftsmen in all the land. Nothing was too good for God. King Solomon was excited and honored to build a dwelling place for God on earth. So he built this exquisite, magnificent temple for the Lord and put in it the very best effort he could. After Solomon completed the construction of the temple, the glory of the Lord filled the house (II Chronicles 5:14).

Are you willing to give God your best? Are you willing to honor him in body and in spirit by caring for your body, God's temple? Do you want the awesome presence of God to dwell richly in your life because He's pleased with His temple?

Let's briefly review what it takes to achieve this goal:

1. Have a positive attitude by focusing on the positive and thinking and speaking positively.
2. Drink plenty of water, at least eight cups per day.
3. Eat natural foods, at least five fruits and vegetables a day, and eat whole grains.
4. Exercise regularly and make activity part of your daily life.
5. Reduce your intake of foods high in fat, sugar, and sodium.
6. Get a fitness partner or someone for support.
7. Get sufficient rest for your body, mind, and spirit.
8. Ultimately, share healthier living and positive experiences with others to create an entire network or support system, and be prepared for battles ahead.

If you incorporate these healthy lifestyle changes into your life, you will lose weight, keep it off, feel better, and look better, too. But it's up to you. How badly do you want it? Are you willing to work for it? Are you willing to make the commitment to do it? Not only will you lose weight; your whole life will change. Even your relationships won't be the same. That is why God told Joshua three times in one chapter to be strong and courageous. It won't always be easy. But you have to be strong, you have to be determined, and you have to have a made up mind that you are going to do what it takes and give God the best effort you can.

To overcome my last trials I had to understand it was up to me. No one was going to do it for me; I was going to do it for myself. So face your fears, face your reason for overeating, discover what is eating you, drop the excess baggage, and strive for success. Just as God gave Joshua the key to obtain his own success, you have the key to success, too. Use the power God gave you. God is not going to come down from heaven, open your mouth, and force you to eat healthier. He is not going to pick you up and make you walk. You have the key, you have the information and the biblical principles, and you *make* it happen. Not only will you be successful, but also God told Joshua he would have "good" success.

I thought all success was good. But with "good" success, you will not succeed by the world's standards; you will be a success in God's eyes. Not only will you get the physical results you want, but in addition you will obtain the inward and eternal blessings that come with true success—joy, peace, happiness, contentment, and your soul will be at rest.

Be prepared. There may be trials that make you feel like the challenge is too much for you to handle. There may be days when you want to totally forget about your health. All of us experience various trials with our spouses, children, jobs, health, finances, or grief from the loss of a loved one. Some of these things can seem devastating, and in many of these incidents the last thing you think about is living healthy. But God wants you to know that no matter how challenging the battle, you don't have to worry. In Joshua 1:9, God covers this, too. He said, *"Have I not commanded you? Be strong and of good courage; do not be afraid, nor be dismayed, for the Lord your God is with you wherever you go."*

No matter what comes up in your life, the Lord is right there to keep you and help you. It doesn't matter where you go or what you go through, you will never be alone in this journey. Joshua and the people of Israel were able to conquer the Promised Land, just as God had promised, by following God's plan for success. Then God gave His people a time of rest, refreshment, and peace when they were able to enjoy the goodness of God and all that He had done for them. As you are eating healthier, losing weight, and feeling better, you will be able to enjoy life as you never have before. So enjoy your results and allow your new attitude to be contagious.

The Bible says, *"For God so loved the world that He gave His only be-gotten Son, that whosoever believes in Him should not perish but have everlasting life."* Jesus died for all of our sins, all of our sicknesses, and for all of our struggles and issues in life. Now we can experience the true "promised land" by having a bright and glorious future in Him in heaven and on earth. For Christ Himself said that He came to give us life and life more abundantly (John 10:10). We can overcome any trial and any temptation through Jesus, who is our greatest example. For the Bible says you can do all things through Christ, who strengthens you (Philippians 4:13). No matter where you have been, what you have done, or how you have neglected your body, you can start over fresh and new. Today is a brand-new day and II Corinthians 5:17 reads, *"Therefore, if anyone is in Christ, he is a new creation; old things have passed away; behold, all things have become new."* You can be anew today and be Fit for God—spirit, soul, and body.

PRAYER

If you have not accepted Christ as your Lord and Savior, say this prayer with me:

Oh God,
I believe you sent Your son Jesus Christ to die for all of my sins. I
believe in my heart that You raised Jesus from the dead so I can

experience an abundant life right here on earth—a life of peace, a life of joy, a life of overcoming any and all obstacles that may come my way. I also believe that through Him my soul will no longer be lost, but I will have eternal life. I thank You for this wonderful gift of salvation and I freely accept it. I ask right now for Jesus to come into my heart, to come into my life, and create something new in me. I want to turn from my old ways of doing things and live a life that's pleasing in Your eyesight. Guide my steps and direct my paths. Give me the strength to do Your will, the strength to care for Your temple, and the strength to let Your light shine so others can see the glory of God in me. Help me to be all that You created me to be, Fit for God—spirit, soul, and body. In Jesus' name. Amen.

Study Scriptures

Matthew 5:16

Let your light so shine before men, that they may see your good works and glorify your Father in heaven.

John 15:16

You did not choose Me, but I chose you and appointed you that you should go and bear fruit, and that your fruit should remain, that whatever you ask the Father in my name He may give you.

John 16:33

These things I have spoken to you, that in Me you may have peace. In the world you will have tribulation; but be of good cheer, I have overcome the world.

ACTIVITIES

1. Make a special effort to share with others this week. You can share some of your healthy lifestyle changes, the results you've gotten, and how you feel. Use your imagination to create some positive experiences for others. You will benefit greatly because you won't be so focused on yourself and obsessed with the scale and the mirror. Before you know it you'll have the results you want while helping others along the way. Start with family and friends until you feel comfortable sharing with others.

2. Develop an action plan. Trials, temptations, and battles will come. Develop a plan of victory to help you overcome such times. By writing in your journal you should have a pretty good idea of what causes you to overeat or not exercise. How will you handle those times of temptations? For instance, if you know you have to face negativity on your job and it causes you stress and temptation, how do you plan on handling it?

I worked in a hectic, high-stress environment with negative people feeding into my spirit daily, but I created a positive and peaceful workspace. I had a magnet on my shelf with a Scripture from the word of God that I read daily. I had a picture of an eagle to remind me that I could soar above any situation. I decorated my desk with plants and flowers to create a lovely, peaceful atmosphere, and my screensaver was a beautiful picture of the beach with waves of water. When I was approached with negativity, I didn't entertain the comment; instead, I reflected on the positive. When my buttons were pushed to the limit, I got up and walked, went in the bathroom and prayed, or called a Christian friend who encouraged me. I saw so many people indulge in food all day long. They had drawers full of snacks or kept bowls of candy on their desks. Many others constantly ran out for a smoke. I developed a plan to overcome wanting to take a piece of chocolate every time I walked past a candy dish. I kept healthy snacks, such as small containers of fruit, in my drawer so I wouldn't get so hungry that I succumbed to eating the chocolate.

3. Create a "New You" List. Replace old habits with new ones. Psychologists and many programs emphasize the importance of replacing bad habits with good habits. For instance, some say if you want to stop smoking, start exercising. When you have one habit, you can't just stop it without replacing the behavior. So it's best to consciously replace it with a positive behavior. This is actually another biblical principle. Ephesians 4:22–24 reads, "*. . . that you put off concerning your former conduct, the old man which grows corrupt according to the deceitful lusts, and be renewed in the spirit of your mind, and that you put on the new man which was created according to God, in true righteousness and holiness.*"

Psychologists say it takes repeating a behavior at least twenty-one times for it to become a habit. So by repeating the new behavior, over a period of time you replace the negative behavior that contributes to poor health. By writing a list of your bad habits and how you plan on replacing them, you are prepared to handle those times of temptation. Here is an example of what you can write in your journal:

"New You" List

Old Behavior (habit)	*New Behavior (to replace old)*
1. Criticizing others	Complimenting others or commenting on their positive qualities
2. Complaining	Focusing on the positive or the good in situations
3. Overeating during meals	Drinking more water during mealtimes and eating more vegetables and salad
4. Late-night snacking	Reading the Bible, praying, or writing in journal
5. Nail-biting, smoking	Exercising, walking, doing stomach crunches

4. Exercise. Continue with your regular exercise routine and make sure you include some activity in your daily life. You can use some of the tips I shared previously on how to stay active. But for this week I also want you to add a new focus to what you do. Most people, whether they want to lose weight or not, are concerned with their stomach. Everybody seems to want a flatter, firmer stomach. Incorporate stomach crunches into your exercise routine in addition to your everyday living routine. For instance, every time you stop at a light while driving, contract (hold in) your stomach and then release when the light turns green. You can also remember to hold in your stomach during the day, and you can even work your stomach muscles at work or while watching television at home. While sitting in a chair, hold on to the armrests. Slowly raise your right knee for a count of four, lower it, then lift the opposite knee. Alternate knees starting with twenty repetitions, increasing them as your muscles get stronger in time. You want to contract your stomach muscles while lifting your knees and release when lowering. And don't forget to breathe. For a more advanced movement, you can lift both knees simultaneously. Make sure you are sitting in a chair with adequate lower back support, and if you feel any unusual pain, listen to your body and stop. If you ride the bus or metro, you don't have to lift your knees, but you can still contract (squeeze) your stomach muscles and release. Remember the key to a flatter, firmer stomach is not just exercising to tone the muscles, but a combination of exercise to strengthen the muscles and aerobics to burn the fat off the top of the stomach.

Scriptures for Success

G od told Joshua the keys to success: reading the Word of God, meditating on the Word, and then doing what it says. When Jesus was tempted by the devil, He used the Word of God to overcome each temptation. The devil was able to tempt Eve because he got her to doubt what God had said. In order to know what God has said for yourself, you need to read and know the Word of God for yourself. Here are some Scriptures for healthy living that can help you overcome those times of temptation and help keep you motivated and encouraged as you strive to take care of your temple. These are Scriptures for a healthy mind, body, and spirit so you can strive to be fit for God.

1. FOR POSITIVE THINKING

Psalm 105:3 Glory in His holy name; let the hearts of those rejoice who seek the Lord!

Psalm 118:24 This is the day the Lord has made; we will rejoice and be glad in it.

Proverbs 23:7 For as he thinks in his heart so is he.

Isaiah 26:3 You will keep him in perfect peace, whose mind is stayed on You because he trusts in You.

Romans 12:2 And do not be conformed to this world, but be transformed by the renewing of your mind, that you may prove what is that good and acceptable and perfect will of God.

II Corinthians 10:4–5 For the weapons of our warfare are not carnal but mighty in God for pulling down strongholds, casting down arguments and every high thing that exalts itself against the knowledge of God, bringing every thought into the captivity to the obedience of Christ . . .

Ephesians 4:22–24 . . . that you put off, concerning your former conduct, the old man which grows corrupt according to the deceitful lusts, and be renewed in the spirit of your mind, and that you put on the new man which was created according to God, in true righteousness and holiness.

Philippians 2:5 Let this mind be in you which was also in Christ Jesus . . .

Philippians 4:4–5 Rejoice in the Lord always. Again I say rejoice! Let your gentleness be known to all men. The Lord is at hand.

Philippians 4:6–7 Be anxious for nothing, but in everything by prayer and supplication, with thanksgiving, let your requests be made known to God; and the peace of God which surpasses all understanding, will guard your hearts and minds through Christ Jesus.

Philippians 4:8 Finally, brethren, whatever things are true, whatever things are noble, whatever things are just, whatever things are pure, whatever things are lovely, whatever things are of good report, if there is any virtue and if there is anything praiseworthy— meditate on these things.

Colossians 3:1–2 If then you were raised with Christ, seek those things which are above, where Christ is, sitting at the right hand of God. Set your mind on things above, not on things on the earth.

2. FOR POSITIVE SPEAKING

Psalm 19:14 Let the words of my mouth and the meditation of my heart be acceptable in Your sight, O Lord, my strength and my Redeemer.

Psalm 34:1 I will bless the Lord at all times; His praise shall continually be in my mouth.

Psalm 34:13 Keep your tongue from evil, and your lips from speaking deceit.

Proverbs 10:31–32 The mouth of the righteous brings forth wisdom, but the perverse tongue will be cut off. The lips of the righteous know what is acceptable, but the mouth of the wicked is perverse.

Proverbs 16:24 Pleasant words are like a honeycomb, sweetness to the soul and health to the bones.

Proverbs 18:21 Death and life are in the power of the tongue, and those who love it will eat its fruit.

Proverbs 18:20 A man's stomach shall be satisfied from the fruit of his mouth; from the produce of his lips he shall be filled.

Matthew 15:18 But those things which proceed out of the mouth come from the heart, and they defile a man.

Romans 4:17 . . . God, who gives life to the dead and calls those things which do not exist as though they did.

Ephesians 4:29 Let no corrupt word proceed out of your mouth, but what is good for necessary edification, that it may impart grace to the hearers.

Colossians 4:6 Let your speech always be with grace, seasoned with salt, that you may know how you ought to answer each one.

James 3:8–10 But no man can tame the tongue. It is an unruly evil, full of deadly poison. With it we bless our God and Father, and with it we curse men, who have been made in the similitude of God. Out of the same mouth proceed blessing and cursing. My brethren, these things ought not be so.

3. FOR A HEALTHY BODY

Deuteronomy 30:19 . . . that I have set before you life and death, blessing and cursing; therefore choose life, that both you and your descendants may live . . .

Psalm 118:17 I shall not die, but live, and declare the works of the Lord.

Psalm 127:1 Unless the Lord builds the house, they labor in vain who build it . . .

Romans 12:1–2 I beseech you therefore, brethren, by the mercies of God, that you present your bodies a living sacrifice, holy, acceptable to God which is your reasonable service. And do not be conformed to this world, but be transformed by the renewing of your mind, that you may prove what is that good and acceptable and perfect will of God.

Romans 13:14 But put on the Lord Jesus Christ, and make no provision for the flesh, to fulfill its lusts.

I Corinthians 3:16–17 Do you not know that you are the temple of God and that the Spirit of God dwells in you? If anyone defiles the temple of God, God will destroy him. For the temple of God is holy, which temple you are.

I Corinthians 6:19–20 Or do you not know that your body is the temple of the Holy Spirit who is in you, whom you have from God, and you are not your own? For you were bought with a price; therefore glorify God in your body and in your spirit, which are God's.

I Corinthians 9:27 But I discipline my body and bring it into subjection, lest, when I have preached to others, I myself should become disqualified.

I Corinthians 10:13 No temptation has overcome you except such is common to man; but God is faithful, who will not allow you to be tempted beyond what you are able, but with the temptation will also make the way of escape, that you may be able to bear it.

I Corinthians 10:31 Therefore, whether you eat or drink, or whatever you do, do all to the glory of God.

Galatians 5:16 I say then: Walk in the Spirit, and you shall not fulfill the lust of the flesh.

Galatians 6:7–9 Do not be deceived, God is not mocked; for whatever a man sows, that he will also reap. For he who sows to his flesh will of the flesh reap corruption, but he who sows to the Spirit will of the Spirit reap everlasting life. And let us not grow weary while doing good, for in due season we shall reap if we do not lose heart.

Ephesians 3:20 To Him who is able to do exceedingly abundantly above all that we ask or think, according to the power that works in us . . .

Philippians 4:13 I can do all things through Christ who strengthens me.

Colossians 3:17 And whatever you do in word or deed, do all in the name of the Lord Jesus, giving thanks to God the Father through Him.

I Thessalonians 5:23 Now may the God of peace Himself sanctify you completely; and may your whole spirit, soul, and body be preserved blameless at the coming of our Lord Jesus Christ.

I Timothy 4:4–5 For every creature of God is good, and nothing is to be refused if it is received with thanksgiving; for it is sanctified by the word of God and prayer.

I Timothy 4:8 For bodily exercise profits a little, but godliness is profitable for all things, having promise of the life that now is and of that which is to come.

Hebrews 12:1–2 Therefore we also, by so great a cloud of witnesses, let us lay aside every weight and the sin which so easily ensnares us, and let us run with endurance the race that is set before us, looking unto Jesus, the author and the finisher of our faith . . .

James 2:20 But do you want to know, O foolish man, that faith without works is dead?

III John 2 Beloved, I pray that you may prosper in all things and be in health, just as your soul prospers.

4. FOR PROPER REST

Genesis 2:2 And on the seventh day God ended His work which He had done, and He rested on the seventh day from all His work which He had done.

Exodus 23:12 Six days you shall do your work, and on the seventh day you shall rest, that your ox and your donkey may rest, and the son of your female servant and the stranger may be refreshed.

Exodus 34:21 Six days you shall work, but on the seventh day you shall rest; in plowing time and harvest time you shall rest.

Psalm 4:8 I will both lie down in peace, and sleep; for You alone, O Lord, make me dwell in safety.

Psalm 23:1–2 The Lord is my Shepherd I shall not want. He makes me lie down in green pastures; He leads me beside the still waters.

Psalm 37:7 Rest in the Lord and wait patiently for Him . . .

Psalm 127:2 It is vain for you to rise up early, to sit up late, to eat bread of sorrows; for so He gives His beloved sleep.

Proverbs 3:24 When you lie down, you will not be afraid; yes, you will lie down and your sleep will be sweet.

Matthew 11:28–30 Come to Me, all you who labor and are heavy laden, and I will give you rest. Take My yoke upon you and learn from Me, for I am gentle and lowly in heart, and your will find rest for your souls. For My yoke is easy and My burden is light.

Mark 6:31 And He said to them, Come aside by yourselves to a deserted place and rest a while.

Hebrews 4:9 There remains therefore a rest for the people of God.

5. For the Word of God

Joshua 1:8 This Book of the Law shall not depart from your mouth, but you shall meditate in it day and night, that you may observe to do according to all that is written in it. For then your will make you way prosperous, and then you will have good success.

Psalm 119:11 Your word I have hidden in my heart, that I might not sin against You.

Psalm 119:105 Your word is a lamp to my feet and a light to my path.

Proverbs 4:20–22 My son, give attention to my words; incline your ear to my sayings. Do not let them depart from your eyes; keep them in the midst of your heart; for they are life to those that find them, and health to all their flesh.

Proverbs 7:1–3 My son, keep my words and treasure my commands within you. Keep my commands and live, and my law as the apple of your eye. Bind them on your fingers; write them on the tablet of your heart.

Isaiah 55:11 So shall My word be that goes forth from My mouth; it shall not return to Me void, but it shall accomplish what I please, and it shall prosper in the thing which I sent it.

John 8:51 Most assuredly, I say to you, if anyone keeps My word he shall never see death.

Romans 10:17 So then faith comes by hearing and hearing by the word of God.

Philippians 2:16 . . . holding fast the word of life, so that I may rejoice in the day of Christ that I have not run in vain or labored in vain.

Colossians 3:16 Let the word of Christ dwell in you richly in all wisdom, teaching and admonishing one another in psalms and hymns and spiritual songs, singing with grace in your hearts to the Lord.

Hebrews 4:12 For the Word of God is living and powerful, and sharper than any two-edged sword, piercing even to the division of soul and spirit, and of joints and marrow, and is a discerner of the thoughts and intents of the heart.

James 1:22 But be doers of the word, and not hearers only, deceiving yourselves.

6. For Prayer

II Chronicles 7:14–15 If My people who are called by My name will humble themselves and pray and seek My face, and turn from their wicked ways, then I will hear from heaven, and will forgive their sin and heal their land. Now My eyes will be open and My ears attentive to prayer made in this place.

Jeremiah 33:3 Call to Me, and I will answer you, and show you great and mighty things which you do not know.

Matthew 6:5 And when you pray, you shall not be like the hypocrites. For they love to pray standing in the synagogues and on the corners of the streets, that they may be seen by men. Assuredly, I say to you, they have their reward.

Matthew 6:6 But you, when you pray, go into your room, and when you have shut the door, pray to your Father who is in the secret place; and your Father who sees in secret will reward you openly.

Matthew 21:13 And He said to them, It is written, My house shall be called a house of prayer . . .

Matthew 26:41 Watch and pray, lest you enter into temptation. The spirit indeed is willing, but the flesh it weak.

Luke 11:2–4 So He said to them, when you pray, say: Our Father in heaven, hallowed be Your name. Your kingdom come. Your will be done on earth as it is in heaven. Give us this day by day our daily bread. And forgive us our sins, for we also forgive everyone who is indebted to us. And do not lead us into temptation, but deliver us from the evil one.

Luke 18:1 Then He spoke a parable to them, that men always ought to pray and not lose heart . . .

Philippians 4:6–7 Be anxious for nothing, but in everything by prayer and supplication, with thanksgiving, let your requests be made known to God; and the peace of God, which surpasses all understanding will guard your hearts and minds through Christ Jesus.

I Thessalonians 5:17 . . . pray without ceasing . . .

James 5:16 . . . and pray for one another, that you may be healed. The effective, fervent prayer of a righteous man avails much.

7. For a Healthy Self-Image (Know who the Bible says you are)

1. *You were made in the image of God.*

Genesis 1:27 So God created man in His own image; in the image of God He created him; male and female He created them.

2. *You are a special treasure to God.*

Deuteronomy 7:6 For you are holy people to the Lord your God; the Lord your God has chosen you to be a people for Himself, a special treasure above all peoples on the face of the earth.

3. *You are fearfully and wonderfully made by God.*

Psalm 139:14 I will praise You, for I am fearfully and wonderfully made; marvelous are Your works, and that my soul knows very well.

4. *God thought of you before you were in your mother's womb.*

Jeremiah 1:5 Before I formed you in the womb I knew you; before you were born I sanctified you; I ordained you a prophet to the nations.

5. *God has a plan for your life.*

Jeremiah 29:11 For I know the thoughts that I think toward you, says the Lord, thoughts of peace and not of evil, to give you a future and a hope.

6. *You have been chosen and ordained by God.*

John 15:16 You did not choose Me, but I chose you and appointed you that you should go and bear fruit, and that your fruit should remain, that whatever you ask the Father in My name He may give you.

7. *You are a child of God.*

Romans 8:16 The Spirit Himself bears witness with our spirit that we are children of God.

8. *You are an heir of God and joint heir with Jesus Christ.*

Romans 8:17 . . . and if children, then heirs—heirs of God and joint heirs with Christ, if indeed we suffer with Him, that we may also be glorified together.

9. *God predestined you to be conformed to the image of His Son.*

Romans 8:29 For whom He foreknew, He also predestined to be conformed to the image of His Son, that He might be the first among many brethren.

10. *You are more than a conqueror through Jesus Christ who loves you.*

Romans 8:37 Yet in all these things we are more than conquerors through Him who loved us.

11. *You are a new creation in Christ.*

II Corinthians 5:17 Therefore, if anyone is in Christ, he is a new creation; old things have passed away; behold, all things have become new.

12. You are an ambassador of God.

II Corinthians 5:20 Now then, we are ambassadors for Christ, as though God were pleading through us; we implore you on Christ's behalf, be reconciled to God.

13. You are a minister of God.

II Corinthians 6:4 But in all things we commend ourselves as ministers of God; in much patience, in tribulation, in needs, in distresses . . .

14. You are Abraham's heir according to the promise.

Galatians 3:29 And if you are Christ's, then you are Abraham's seed, and heirs according to the promise.

15. You were chosen by God before the foundation of the world.

Ephesians 1:4 . . . just as He chose us in Him before the foundation of the world, that we would be holy and without blame before Him in love . . .

16. You are the adopted of God by Jesus Christ to Himself.

Ephesians 1:5 Having predestined us to adoption as sons by Jesus Christ to Himself, according to the good pleasure of His will . . .

17. You are a member of the household of God and a dwelling place for God.

Ephesians 2:19, 22 Now, therefore, you are no longer strangers and foreigners, but fellow citizens with the saints and members of the household of God . . . in whom the whole building, being fitted together, grows into a holy temple in the Lord, in whom you also are being built together for a dwelling place of God in the Spirit.

18. You are cherished by God.

Ephesians 5:29 For no one ever hated his own flesh, but nourishes it and cherishes it, just as the Lord does the church.

19. You are a chosen generation and a royal priesthood.

I Peter 2:9 But you are a chosen generation, a royal priesthood, a holy nation, His own special people, that you may proclaim the praises of Him who called you out of darkness into His marvelous light . . .

20. You are the elect of God.

Colossians 3:12 Therefore, as the elect of God, holy and beloved, put on tender mercies, kindness, humility, meekness, long-suffering . . .

21. You are the beloved of God.

II Thessalonians 2:13 But we are bound to give thanks to God always for you, brethren beloved by the Lord, because God from the beginning chose you for salvation through sanctification by the Spirit and belief in the truth, to which He called you by our gospel, for the obtaining of the glory of our Lord Jesus Christ . . .

22. One day you will be just like Christ.

I John 3:2 Beloved, now we are children of God; and it has not yet been revealed what we shall be, but we know that when He is revealed, we shall be like Him, for we shall see Him as He is.

23. You are a king and a priest of God.

Revelation 1:5–6 . . . and from Jesus Christ, the faithful witness, the firstborn from the dead, and the ruler over the kings of the earth. To Him who loved us and washed us from our sins in His own blood, and has made us kings and priests to His God and Father, to Him be glory.

24. You are so loved by God that He sent Jesus Christ to die for your sins.

John 3:16 For God so loved the world that He gave His only be-gotten Son, that whosoever believes in Him should not perish but have everlasting life.

25. *You are so loved by God that no sin, fault, mistake, problem or tribulation can stop God from loving you.*

Romans 8:38 For I am persuaded that neither death nor life, nor angels nor principalities nor power, nor things present nor things to come, nor height nor depth, nor any created thing shall be able to separate us from the love of God which is in Christ Jesus our Lord.

About the Author

La Vita Weaver has shared health and fitness around the world as the cohost of Trinity Broadcast Network's (TBN's) Christian fitness show *TotaLee Fit*. She is also the producer and host of the award-winning local cable health and fitness show *Eternally Fit*. As a mother of three who at her heaviest weighed two hundred pounds, she lost weight and overcame bingeing and depression through her spiritually based fitness program. As a certified personal trainer and fitness counselor with over ten years' experience in the physical fitness industry and as an ordained minister, she inspires others to live healthier lives, heal spiritually, and experience an abundant life in Christ through Fit for God workshops and seminars. She is also the originator of Hallelujah! Aerobics for Body and Spirit—the first spiritually based aerobic program of its kind. La Vita's success story was aired on TBN's *Praise the Lord* and *The 700 Club,* and was in *Shape, Heart and Soul,* and *Excellence* magazines. For more information about the ministry or Christian aerobic videos, visit fitforgod.net or contact Fit for God Ministries, P.O. Box 3473, Capitol Heights, MD 20791, tel. (301) 901-3013.